THE

21-Day
Del Mar Diet

Other books in this series by Dr. Know•How Publications:

The Complete Del Mar Diet — 0-9609040-1-8
The 21 Day Del Mar Diet — 0-9609040-2-6
Nutritional Common Sense — 0-9609060-2-7
Nutritional Healing — 0-9609050-8-5
Tips for Feeling Tops — 0-9609040-3-4
Countdown to Success — 0-9609040-4-2
Mending Your Emotional Wounds — 0-9609040-5-0
The Meltzer Wellness Program — 0-9609040-6-9

ISBN: 0-9609040-1-8

First printing 1982

THE
21-Day
Del Mar Diet

By BARNET MELTZER, M.D.

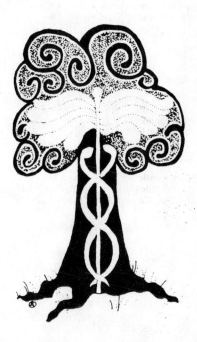

Dr. Know•How Publications

ACKNOWLEDGMENTS

The author gratefully acknowledges his many patients and friends, that have taught him the meaning of nutritional healing. Special thanks go to my Mother and Father. I dearly appreciate the help from June, Art, Liz, Hyiah, Harold, Gina, and Jan for their support. I want to also acknowledge Tim Donohue, for his penetrating insight. Actually, this book is only possible because of all the beautiful people in my life.

TABLE OF CONTENTS
THE 21-DAY DEL MAR DIET

INTRODUCTION

Another book on weight loss? Another diet fad? We need another book on diet like the bearded lady needs another hair on her face. No, this is not just another book. This is the ultimate nutrition book. This is the definitive book on diet. No other book is needed.

Your search for that right and perfect diet is over. It is just that simple. The Del Mar Diet is conclusive. It precisely defines exactly what you need to know about your optimal diet. It is fully developed so that you can use the program to feel your best or to lose burdensome weight.

I call it the Del Mar Diet. Although its origins were at the Bronx High School of Science in New York City, at the University of Pennsylvania in Philadelphia, on the beaches in Ft. Lauderdale, in the emerald-green mountains of South America, and at the UCLA Medical Center, it reached its fruition in Del Mar, California. I have had a remarkable success story with my patients utilizing this diet to enrich their health. Feeling great, attaining sexual virility and achieving longevity are the dividends of the plan.

I am not going to belabor all that has been written before. I'm going to direct you and explain to you, and you will do the rest. I'm not going to request your cooperation; you ultimately must want to achieve that fit and trim look. You and only you must take charge and modify your lifestyle to get there. Are you sick and tired of being sick and tired? Are unpleasant and unhealthy feelings of being out of shape or overweight plaguing you? Then this is the book for you.

The 21 Day Del Mar Diet is divided into 3 segments:

WEEK 1: *The Cleansing Diet.*

WEEK 2: *The Detoxification Diet.*

WEEK 3: *The Maintenance Diet.*

After the first three weeks you follow the unique rhythm method of this program.

Keep in mind that your stamina, appearance and your strength reflect the quality of your diet. The Del Mar Diet keeps you looking your very best. Added benefits include a strong heart, a mighty body, and a longer life. The program touches all of you.

The essence of the diet is to guarantee maximum individual performance at home, at work, or at play. When you are sustaining high level wellness, it is no accident. You know what you are doing.

TAKE IT TO THE LIMIT

The Diet has a number of interesting features. The fundamental attributes are:

- It's **workability:** The Del Mar Diet is practical and, above all, it works!

- **Reliability:** The Del Mar Nutritional Program is the basis for longevity and wellness for thousands of patients.

- The nutritional **balance** inherent in the plan.

- Its natural **rhythm:** The rhythm method of the cleansing and detoxification diets cleans out the toxins in your system, and washes out the poisons from your body fluids. This sharpens up the cutting edge of your metabolic machinery. This service prevents the accumulation of grease and grime. The result is that your tissues function well.

- **Permanent weight loss:** Dieters can lose as much as 15-21 pounds in the first three weeks. You can stop counting calories on a scale. The Maintenance Diet is a built-in support system. You enjoy your food, while keeping yourself fit and trim at your ideal weight.

- Its **safety:** The simple, yet specific, food instructions assure you an abundance of quality food nutrients. Guidelines show you how to get enough protein without having to eat meat. Everything has been worked out for you. You can stop worrying about your health.

- **Sound Eating Habits:** Timely relaxed undereating habits are the building blocks of the diet. You learn the basics about how to eat your food in order to maximize your assimilation of essential life·giving nutrients.

- **Its power to prevent disease:** The Diet naturally prevents high blood pressure, diabetes, arthritis, and other degenerative illnesses from attacking your body.

- **Lasting benefits:** Good health, endless energy, sexual vigor, mental alertness, and a clear sense of overall well-being.

- **Effective food combining:** To assure sound digestion and efficient absorption of essential food nutrients.

- **Variety and Excitement:** Highly nutritious food prepared to satisfy your palate, is a well established health secret of this diet.

— WHAT ARE YOU WAITING FOR? —

The time has come to convert talk into action, and ideas into experience. In the upcoming chapters, you learn to:

- *Eat Right.*
- *Balance your diet.*
- *Diet to lose weight permanently.*
- *Eat for food power:* To select, combine, and prepare your food correctly.
- *Organize your health food kitchen.*
- *Map out your breakfast, lunch, and dinner.*
- *Take the right nutritional supplements to stay young in mind and body.*

With the digestive aid of the Del Mar Diet, you learn how to take control of your own life. Remember that your strategy must ultimately be integrated and coordinated into what you do every day. Go forward, and get off the treadmill of *your* life? The 21 Day Del Mar Diet will pave your way to success.

PREFACE

Many years ago in the City of Brotherly Love, there was a man writhing in pain, who appeared in the emergency room coughing up rusty sputum. It was 3:15 a.m. in the black of the night. Just moments before he arrived, I was enjoying the illusion that after starting the intravenous antibiotic drip on Mrs. Murphy, I was free to get some shuteye. I had just fallen asleep in the top bunk of the doctors' sleeping quarters when I was jarred awake by the deep, heavy voice of the head nurse.

"Dr. Meltzer, I just admitted a very sick patient with left-sided chest pain. His vital signs are stable, except for his temperature. It is 103.4°. Hurry on over."

"I'll be right down," I said as I looked around in the darkness for my clothes. As the ranking fourth year medical student, I was the student physician covering all admissions to ward 7 East until the sun came up. Those long nights were some of the first real opportunities I had to play doctor. That particular morning I knew I couldn't stop the sun from rising, and I wouldn't be back to bed. With my eyes half open, I scurried down the poorly lit corridors to the emergency room.

I diagnosed the patient, Leroy, a 55-year-old alcoholic diabetic, as having a bad case of pneumonia. I admitted him to the medical ward and was responsible to write the orders for the nursing staff to follow. You see, orders were written by the admitting M.D. in a big green looseleaf at the nursing station with the patient's name on it. After you wrote your orders, you placed the chart back into a lazy susan and flagged them for the nurses' attention.

I wrote orders for Leroy to have plenty of bed rest and to have his blood pressure, pulse, temperature, and respirations (his vital signs) checked every 20 minutes. I started him on a loading dose of penicillin, some pain medication, and instructed the nurses to put Leroy through some vigorous coughing exercises to clean out his pulmonary toilet. I wrote these orders as a matter of routine.

While accompanying Leroy on the stretcher up the elevator, he told me he was hungry. He wanted to know what he could eat. How was I supposed to know? After all, I was just the doctor. Nutrition had only been mentioned a few times in passing when I was a third year medical student. So I wrote the popular diet order that I saw the senior resident physicians write — "regular diet." This meant that Leroy could eat whatever he wanted to. And he did. To associate Leroy's eating habits with the onset, cause, or course of his illness was not within the scope of my medical knowledge at that time.

Whenever the subject came up of what was the right diet to prescribe, I had two choices. I could always consult the hospital staff dietician. They were usually very friendly and very cooperative. The traditional nutritionists limited their association of poor nutrition to beri-beri, scurvy, pellagra, sunken eyeballs, wasted extremeties, and swollen abdomens. There was only one difficulty with them. Literally, food was their business. They were usually 50 to 80 pounds too heavy. By and large, they suffered with the *malnutrition of overconsumption.* Frankly, the majority of the staff dieticians were just too overweight for me to trust their academic words of wisdom. The doctors had less training in nutrition than the dieticians. They admittedly were not in the position to answer my nutritional questions.

Thankfully, there was one other place to turn. My grandmother's folklorish chicken-vegetable soup remedy. Since my grandma had eaten more meals at age 80 than anyone else in my family, she was my nutritional consultant. She advised me to give Leroy a glass of warm milk with some sweetened aspirin and a cherry-flavored cough syrup three times a day. Within 36 hours of admission, Leroy was asking his family to bring him his favorite foods. He felt most comfortable resuming his normal dietary consumption of beef and pastries.

I soon found it easier to ignore my patients' nutritional needs than to try to meet them. I could get my medical degree without having to really know anything about nutrition. I was a good student. I regurgitated what "they" wanted to hear. I buried myself in the dry medical textbooks, devouring fact after fact that I hoped some day would come in handy. I got straight A's in medicine, surgery, pediatrics, obstetrics, gynecology, and, of necessity, tabled my concerns about nutrition and nutritional therapy until after I graduated from medical school.

THE TURNING POINT

My interest in human nutrition really began to pick up after my medical school years. In the springtime of 1971, I was flying high as an up-and-coming surgical resident at the University of California in San Diego. A close friend of mine invited me to go along to a health symposium at the downtown convention center. The podium was filled with eminent speakers. One noted physician was speaking about the benefits of a balanced diet.

In those days a balanced diet was *in*. You see, it was the

beginning of the consumer movement towards questioning our standard nutritional values. Every time the word 'balanced' was mentioned, it brought down the house with applause.

After the fifteenth time the speaker mentioned the term 'balanced diet,' I can vividly remember what transpired. I started to feel a bit uneasy. My pulse quickened. I thought to myself either I was the dumbest person in the whole convention hall, or I'm the only one to have the guts to ask. I respectfully stood up. I raised my hand. My words reverberated throughout the El Cortez Hotel. "Mr. Speaker, I beg your pardon. My name is Barnet G. Meltzer. I am a surgical resident at the University of California. Please enlighten me. *What exactly do you mean by a balanced diet?*"

"A balanced diet is, you know, well, er, it's usually umm, let's see, hmm, I think, you know, er, it's usually, well let's see, maybe. . . . Everybody knows what a balanced diet is . . . ah . . . um . . . a balanced diet is . . . ahh. . . ." Well, after much humming and hawing, the speaker came right to the point. "*A balanced diet is a balanced diet.*" After a short discussion, I realized that there was much confusion. There was absolutely no consensus as to what were the ingredients of a balanced diet.

I looked to that evening's lecture as one of the turning points in my life. That night I strengthened my resolve and made up my mind to determine exactly what constitutes a balanced diet. I spent the next 12 years learning the secrets of man's optimal diet. And what I found out was so drastically different than what I was led to believe. I have never been the same. It was incredible. I have treated thousands of patients in my office in Southern California. I did a nutritional research tour of Mexico and Central America. I spent nearly three years on horseback riding through the wilds of the South American Andes studying the diets of very sheltered, primitive peoples. I returned to my beloved California. There was no doubt about it.

MAN'S OPTIMAL DIET IS RICH IN:

- **Fresh fruits.**
- **Fresh raw vegetables.**
- **The vegetable proteins of staple whole grains and legumes.**

Big business, TV commercials, restaurants, magazine and newspaper food features encourage the consumption of dangerous toxic devitalized foods. I witnessed the No. 1 nutritional deficiency in South America to be *under*consumption malnutrition. I realized that *over*consumption malnutrition was truly the No. 1 nutritional deficiency in the United States. It was the direct result of overeating poor-quality preservative-rich foods.

This suicidal nutritional condition is intimately related to the menancing level of inertia and mediocrity threatening our very lifestyles. Simply take a look at your level of stress, your degree of sexual satisfaction, your level of emotional fulfillment or happiness, or your blood pressure, your triglyceride level, your cholesterol, or your weight to know what long-term effects your present dietary lifestyle has created. You are what you choose to eat. Your relationship with your diet has the same meaningful connection as does the ripened fruit growing from a healthy tree. Let me put the cards on the table, you can play them, or request a new deal.

THE COMPLETE
21-Day
Del Mar Diet

1: THE DEL MAR DIET:
Your Optimal Diet

Everybody wants to look good and feel great. The fact of the matter is that when you eat right you feel well. Why not take control of your life. Eating your way to wellness is the solution. Following a diet that is optimal for you is the natural place to start.

Your optimal diet is simple and efficient. It *simply* provides your mental, physical, emotional, and spiritual bodies with the right food nutrients at the cellular level. It *efficiently* creates high-level positive energy for the tissues in your body to function well. Your optimal diet is the staff of life. *It feeds your mind, sustains your body, and nourishes your spirit.* It also illuminates your emotions. To keep fit and be happy you *need* the finest grade of nutritional fuel.

The acid test of an optimal diet is that it works so well that your metabolic machinery exercises its incredible healing powers with silent, yet piercingly effective, harmonious orchestration. That is, you love, walk, talk, play, work, exercise, sleep, eat, and make love effortlessly.

In essence, the purpose of your optimal diet is to sustain lasting wellness.

THE DEL MAR DIET IS YOUR OPTIMAL DIET

The Del Mar Diet is a proven winner. It satisfies all the requirements for an optimal diet: it is practical, reliable, tasty and appetizing. It takes into consideration your social life, your habits, your sex life and your life style as well as your nutritional needs. Fundamentally, it is a natural Hi·Lite Hi·Enzyme Diet. Here is how it works.

The Del Mar Diet is a Light Diet. Hi·Lite food is pure wholesome food free of artificial preservatives and additives. It is the product of plenty of good air and natural sunshine. That is why it is rich in nutritional electricity. Hi·Lite nutrition is pregnant with vital nutrients and vibrant life force. This super·nutrition is derived from being *"naturally enriched"* with maturing vitamins, minerals and other essential micronutrients. This gives it lots of power. The better the soil, the more punch to its Lite·force.

Hi·Lite food is good for you. It gives you a life time of healthy, fresh Hi·Life food. It also gets you high. The Del Mar Diet provides you with the life-giving current that keeps the condition of your body battery in fine running order. This Diet makes you tough. Healthy Hi·Lite food power also gives you the strength to see the Light in your life.

Hi·Lite food is stacked with natural enzymes. You can be certain that the most superior foods are Hi-Enzymes foods. Hi-Enzyme foods are alive. The Enzymes are the Life·Giving·Principles. They are beneficial, organic, chemical messengers. They carry the Universal Life·Giving·Nutrients that transform the living cells in your whole body into a bio·chemical state of total nourishment.

WHAT ARE THE BEST FOODS TO EAT?

Nature's hi·enzyme foods, rich in Light·force are the best foods to eat. They offer you the benefits of high quality, top of the line nutrition without toxic side effects.

Therefore your optimal diet is rich in:

> * *Ripened fresh fruits, in season.*
> * *Living fresh raw vegetables.*
> * *Fresh living fruit and vegetable juices.*
> * *Sprouted seeds and grains.*
> * *Natural high quality vegetable protein of whole grains and legumes, such as soybeans, lentils, dried peas, and beans. Small amounts of natural oils offered in nuts and seeds are essential to lubricate your delicate, intricate, sensitive biological systems.*

Hi·Enzyme natural foods nourish your cells to their highest level of intelligence. And, your cells are quite intelligent. They can heal, change, adapt, accept or reject, think, feel, act, create and transform. They have a will of their own. Their fate is up to you. Through your thoughts, feelings and actions, you choose *your* own nutritional evolution.

It is a simple truth that processed, refined, devitalized, packaged, convenient food has been stripped of its Light·force. Whether it be long or short-term, eating food with a deficiency of fundamental life-giving enzymatic principles causes biochemical imbalance. This leads to body breakdown. A lower grade of nutritional fuel is responsible for the "Twilight Zone"** of relative nutritional deficiencies.

You deserve the best. Why not choose to be well-nourished? Your health, your longevity, your sex life, and your happiness all depend on the ability of your mind and body to stay in excellent running condition at all times. Make the break today. *COMMIT YOURSELF TO CHOOSING THE HIGHEST QUALITY HI·ENZYME HI·LITE NUTRITIONAL FUEL.*

**See page 27

STRIKE A BALANCE

On purpose, your optimal diet balances out your body chemistry. It brings you into internal balance. In sticking to the proper food combinations the Del Mar diet brings you into harmony with your emotional and physiological needs. Your body gets trim and strong and your moods get stabilized. Your spirit comes alive and your mental attitude shines in the Light.

The balance in the Del Mar Diet keeps the engines of your mind churning. It provides an abundant reservoir of energy so you can function very well. The exceptional quality of the Del Mar Diet also feeds your emotional and spiritual wellness.

How you begin to feel is the magic of the program. Balancing the chemistry in your cells and bodily fluids turns on your very own orderly enzymatic vital life energies. As you Lighten up, your whole being comes alive! In turn, this leads to greater **Strength** and further **Balance**.

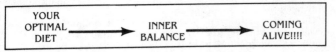

YOUR OPTIMAL DIET ——→ INNER BALANCE ——→ COMING ALIVE!!!!

THE DEL MAR DIET WORKS!
KEEP TO THE RHYTHM

What naturally follows when you eat right is that you experience, maybe for the first time in your adult life, the sensational thrill of being fully alive. How is it that one diet can get you balanced and further keep you that way? The secret lies in the **rhythm method** of the Del Mar Diet. The program is actually a series of diets. The complete Del Mar Diet is made up of a Cleansing, Detoxification, and Maintenance Diet. A juice fasting program is also part of your Detoxification routine.

Your search for the right diet is over. Knowing how and when to cleanse, detoxify, juice fast or maintain is what keeps you well. This is all you have to know.

- **The Cleansing Diet:** To cleanse your body, clarify your mind, brighten up your spirit, and get rid of the accumulated poisons of modern day living.

- **The Detoxification Diet:** To strengthen your immune system and purge your body of deep-seated poisons.

- **The Maintenance Diet:** To nourish your whole being to wellness.

- **The Fasting Program:** To keep your metabolism rejuvenated and your weight under control.

The lifetime, *"Keep-it-Off"* Del Mar Permanent weight loss program is a variation on the above theme. Knowing how and when to Cleanse, Detoxify and Juice Fast makes it easy to maintain your ideal weight.

HOW TO USE THE PROGRAM

The basic 21 Day Del Mar Diet is divided into three weeks.

WEEK 1: *Nutritional Cleansing:* to lighten up your life

WEEK 2: *Nutritional Detoxification:* to purge out bodily poisons

WEEK 3: *Nutritional Maintenance:* to balance out your body chemistry

The Del Mar Diet is for everyone. Teenagers, adults, and senior citizens can all do very well. Children under 14 and pregnant women only need the Maintenance Plan.

Those of you in good health, looking for optimal health, are rewarded by sticking to the 21 day plan. Invariably you feel terrific. For most, you lose 7-10 pounds in the first two weeks. By the end of three weeks you shed 10-15 pounds. You see, the Maintenance Diet levels you off, and keeps it off. Depending upon how much you exercise, you can sometimes lose 20 pounds or more. In any event, wellness and not just losing unsightly pounds is the focus for your program.

It is very interesting that as you break down the poisons, folks in mediocre health may experience some fatigue or vague symptoms of withdrawal. This usually goes away by the end of the Cleansing Diet or shortly after you begin week two Detox. See the risks of the Cleansing Diet page 15 for details. Individuals in poor health, or those who suffer with functional hypoglycemia, diabetes, cancer and other metabolic disturbances can follow the 21 Day Del Mar Diet with a few modest modifications. In these cases, it is well advised that you be under the supervision of your family doctor.

For those of you that need to lose more than 15 pounds, you have a weight problem. Do something about it. Begin with the easy to follow, "Rapid, 21 day" weight loss segment of the program. "See Chapter 8, page 143." It is very close to the original 21 Day Del Mar Diet. It differs because it has more juice fasting, and follows through with a Take · Charge · Keep · Slim Maintenance Diet.

WHAT HAPPENS AFTER 21 DAYS?

Thanks for asking. There is something more you need to know about the Del Mar Diet. The balance of nature is its teacher.

To be well and stay that way you have to keep in balance with the natural changes in the climate and weather in your environment. Nature is always changing. And so are you. A great deal of your health has to do with keeping abreast with the natural changes taking place as the seasons change. When you do it right, it is called being in tune with nature.

Optimal health is actually the ability to stay well in spite of the inevitable changes in the weather. Have you ever noticed how most everyone at work or at school is coming down with a "what's going around virus" at the very time there is a change in the season. That is where the term "under the weather" comes from. It is the responsibility of your optimal diet to sustain your natural rhythm so you're not thrown off course. Who can afford the loss of time from work or play?

THE RHYTHM METHOD OF THE DEL MAR DIET

The rhyme and reason of the Del Mar Diet is to keep you centered. The focus is to stay in balance with the seasonal changes. To do this the Del Mar Diet is a quarterly plan based on the four seasons. Within each season the balance and nutritional support rotates around the timing of your Cleansing, Detox, Maintenance and Juice Fasting Plan.

SEASONAL TIMING COUNTS

The prescription of the Del Mar nutritional program looks like this. Within each 90 day period you follow:

1. **A BALANCED MAINTENANCE DIET** for approximately 75-85% of the time.

2. **CLEANSING, DETOXIFICATION, OR FASTING DIETS** are the nutritional therapy of choice for approximately 15-25% of the days.

The frequency and duration of the Del Mar Cleansing, Detoxification, and Fasting protocols are prescribed to keep you leveled off and equalized.

I. AT EACH EQUINOX:
Practice 5 days on the *Del Mar Cleansing Diet.* It is best to begin 10 days before each seasonal change (equinox). The seasonal cleansings are as follows:

 • Spring seasonal cleansing 7-10 days before March 20-22 (mark your calendar on March 10)
 • Summer seasonal cleansing 7-10 days before June 20-22 (mark your calendar on June 10)
 • Autumn seasonal cleansing 7-10 days before September 20-22 (mark your calendar on September 10)
 • Winter seasonal cleansing 7-10 days before December 20-22 (mark your calendar on December 10)

II. AT THE MIDSEASON:
Practice 5 days on the *Del Mar Detoxification Diet.* Start at the *midway point* between the seasonal changes. Therefore, the mid-seasonal detoxification is as follows:

 • Spring mid-seasonal detoxification the first week in May.
 • Summer mid-seasonal detoxification the first week in August.
 • Autumn mid-seasonal detoxification the first week in November.
 • Winter mid-seasonal detoxification the first week in February.

III. JUICE FAST 1 DAY A WEEK:
Choose the first working day of each week to juice it. After 2 years on the Del Mar Diet juice fasting can be substituted for the cleansing and detoxification diets at the seasonal and mid-seasonal junctures. Then, cleanse and detoxify for 5 days respectively after your seasonal and mid-seasonal juice fasting.

RHYTHMIC BLUEPRINT FOR YOUR SEASONAL DEL MAR DIET

SPRING EQUINOX — March 20*			SUMMER EQUINOX — June 20*		
	3/20-4/30	Maintenance Diet — juice fast 1 day a week		6/20-7/31	Maintenance Diet — juice fast 1 day a week
MID-SEASONAL DETOXIFI-CATION	5/1-5/5	Detoxification Diet	MID-SEASONAL DETOXIFI-CATION	8/1-8/5	Detoxification Diet
	5/6-6/9	Maintenance Diet — juice fast 1 day a week		8/6-9/9	Maintenance Diet — juice fast 1 day a week
SEASONAL CLEANSING	6/10-6/15	Cleansing Diet	SEASONAL CLEANSING	9/10-9/15	Cleansing Diet
	6/16-6/19	Maintenance Diet		9/16-9/19	Maintenance Diet
AUTUMNAL EQUINOX — Sept. 20*			WINTER EQUINOX — December 20*		
	9/20-10/31	Maintenance Diet — juice fast 1 day a week		12/20-1/31	Maintenance Diet — juice fast 1 day a week
MID-SEASONAL DETOXIFI-CATION	11/1-11/5	Detoxification Diet	MID-SEASONAL DETOXIFI-CATION	2/1-2/5	Detoxification Diet
	11/6-12/9	Maintenance Diet — juice fast 1 day a week		2/6-3/9	Maintenance Diet — juice fast 1 day a week
SEASONAL CLEANSING	12/10-12/15	Cleansing Diet	SEASONAL CLEANSING	3/10-3/15	Cleansing Diet
	12/16-12/19	Maintenance Diet		3/16-3/19	Maintenance Diet

You can do the first 21 Days whenever you want. And then keep up the beat. In Light of your quarterly cleansing, it is best to begin the basic 21 Day Plan right at the start, or at the middle of a new season.

Once you have completed the initial 21 Days, plug into the natural rhythm of the diet. In effect, then, the Del Mar Diet is based upon the fundamentals principle of preventative medicine: keep yourself balanced to stay well. In harmony with yourself, you stand the most favorable chance to keep in harmony with your changing environment. The truth is that when you are well nourished you can stay in charge of *your* life. Your optimal diet gives you the adaptability to stay internally balanced with the changing forces in the world around you.

TAKE CONTROL TO GET THE POWER

The natural hi-enzyme diets of Hi·Lite Cleansing, Detoxification, Maintenance, and juice fasting, working in harmony with the seasonal changes is your optimal diet. By adhering to the natural rhythm of quarterly cleansing and mid-seasonal detoxification you assume ground control power and gain control of your life. It is the unique food combinations and timing of this Del Mar diet that gives you the power to:

- *Cleanse* destructive toxins from the blood and the lymph to enhance the healing powers of the circulation.

- *Purify* the mind and emotions. Costly impurities from the central nervous system and the ductless glands are removed in exchange for a positive mental attitude and inner happiness. This allows for your positive feelings and emotions to flow without the obstructions of a toxic bodily physiology.

- *Detoxify* poisoned and overworked vital organs, such as liver, kidneys, and intestines, and make room for positive life-giving nutrients.

- *Activate* the body's natural detoxifying powers to render noxious wastes and poisons harmless.

- *Eliminate* harmful sediment, plaque, wastes, deposits, and toxins from the body.

- *Arrest* uncalled for bodily decay and degeneration.

- *Restore* nourishment to worn out nerves and exhausted glands.

- *Revitalize* the sex glands.

- *Rejuvenate* the spirit.

- *Elevate* your consciousness.

- *Create* optimal super · nutrition.

- *Maintain* optimal nourishment.

- *Sustain* optimal nourishment.

THE DEL MAR MAINTENANCE DIET
IS THE NEW AGE DIET

The principle diet of the Del Mar Nutritional program is a balanced Hi·Lite maintenance diet. This diet is the optimal maintenance diet for man in his present evolution. Why? Because it provides a truly balanced relationship between carbohydrates, proteins, and fats. The essence of this fresh natural diet is:

- *high* in natural hi-enzyme Carbohydrates,
- *moderate* in highly spirited Vegetable Protein, and
- *low* in hi-enzyme natural Fats.

NEW AGE FOOD GROUPING
CHART I

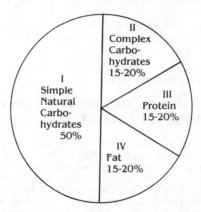

I. *Simple Natural Carbohydrates* (fresh fruits, fresh vegetables, and fresh natural juices) — 50%.

II. *Whole Complex Carbohydrates* (whole grain breads, cereals, and natural starches) — 15-20%.

III. *High-quality Proteins* — 15-20%.

IV. *Natural Fats* — 15-20%.

There are 11 main criteria that harmoniously blend together to create the experience of the balanced maintenance diet. The ingredients provide the *right amount* and the *right proportions* of:

1. *High quality simple natural carbohydrates:* 50% of the Optimal Maintenance Diet (O.M.D.).

2. *Whole complex carbohydrates:* 15-20% of the O.M.D.

3. *High-quality protein:* 15-20% of the O.M.D.

4. *Vegetable to animal protein:* The ratio of vegetable to animal protein is of the utmost importance. At least 70% and as much as 85% (and in some individuals up to 100%) as vegetable protein.

5. *Natural fats:* 15-20%.

6. *Natural unsaturated to saturated fats:* 2/3 of the total fat intake of the optimal maintenance diet is unsaturated fatty acids.

7. *Minerals and vitamins:* Provided by the balanced maintenance diet in substantial quantities to insure optimal nutrition.

8. *Raw to cooked foods:* At least 50% of the diet as fresh, raw, living food.

9. *Alkaline to acid balance:* A ratio of 3 parts alkaline to 2 parts acid (3:2). For some individuals as much as 2:1 alkaline to acid.

10. *Dietary fiber:* At least 25 gms. daily.

11. *Color balance:* The optimal maintenance diet is creatively aesthetic and visually appealing.

TAKE A STAND ON THE FOODS MOST COMMONLY AVAILABLE

When you eat the Right foods in the Right proportions, you THRIVE. You are not eating too much or too little of any vital nutrient. You avoid harmful, inferior quality fuel. Nutritional excess, nutritive abuses, and low quality toxic fuel are the most common· trigger causes of fatigue, mental wasting, anxiety, and depression. Nutritional imbalance throws you into the nutritional twilight zone.*

SUGAR: Any amount of table sugar is too much. Excess white sugar creates an inefficient, unstable, and faulty metabolism. Refined sugars weaken your adrenal glands, overtax your nerves, and deplete B vitamins. The deficiency state of functional hypoglycemia is often the result.

WHITE FLOUR: Processed, refined (bleached or unbleached) white flour is harmful to your health. White bread has no natural enzyme nutritive value. Eating white bread clogs your digestive track. Eating too much bread puts on weight in the wrong places.

SALT: Salt in your diet damages your kidneys. It has destructive effects on your stomach as well. Excess salt makes you high risk for high blood pressure. Do not salt your food.

*See page 27

MEATS: AVOID MEAT PROTEIN. Red meat is loaded with synthetic chemicals. Meat is a toxic fuel that fills you up artificially and gives you a drugged hyped-up energy level. Beef protein is obstructive. It hurts your pancreas. Red meat protein consumption results in heavy accumulation of acid residue toxins in the body. This damages nerves and especially joints. Meat has been cited as a risk factor to the increased incidence in rectal and colon cancer. Over-Proteinzation, or eating more animal protein than you need, whether it be meat, fish, or chicken, is a negative cultural phenomenon.

FATS: High fat levels clog the circulation. They are major contributory risk factors for hardening of the arteries, diabetes, and obesity. Excess fat in your diet increase your vulnerability to breast cancer, cancer of the uterus, as well as gall bladder cancer and other malignancies. Too much meat or dairy is a common nutritional turn-over. Animal fats, in particular meat and lard are high in cholesterol. They have a molesting influence on your hormonal balance. Grease prematurely rusts your system.

REFINED CARBOHYDRATES: White rice impairs your liver's ability to be the detoxifying machine that it can be. Avoid sweets, and artificially sweetened foods.

SOFT DRINKS: A cultural rip-off, nutritionally. They contain hidden caffeine, sugar, and artificial chemicals.

MILK: The most exaggerated food in the world for adults and teen-agers. Milk is very mucus forming. Pasteurized milk overstimulates the upper respiratory passages, ears, nose, throat, sinuses, and the lungs to oversecrete. Pasteurized milk allergies are common. Digestive gland function and assimilation is also compromised from excessive mucus formation.

CAFFEINE: Caffeinism is a social ritual. Overstimulation to the nerves, adrenals, and heart is hazardous to your well-being. Headaches and breast lumps are common.

You are smart to avoid the excess of any nutrient that increases your risk to suffer with a diet-related deficiency. Why do I make such a fuss over these frequently-advertised easy access food items? Because they have a corrosive effect on the integrity of your digestive enzymes. The net effect of this pernicious influence is incomplete assimilation of vital life-giving nutrients.

With the help of your optimal diet, your body will learn to assimilate your food well. This means that your mind opens, body solidifies, emotions prosper, and spirit reaches out. It also suggests that you get what you need from what you choose to eat. Your optimal diet is a very powerful form of preventive medicine. When your optimal diet is well assimilated, you can completely satisfy the appetites of your whole body.

Eating your way to wellness is an orderly, natural process. It naturally evolves from responsible nutritional decision making.

Nevertheless, adolescent teenagers and many on-the-go employees often fall victim to eating what is convenient . . . plenty of sweets, fats, soft drinks, delicatessen meats, chemically processed acid-forming beef, fried chicken, and shellfish. Or, you start missing meals because you are rushed. On-the-go nutrition results in nutritional imbalance because of inferior assimilation of minerals, vitamins, and vegetable proteins. Avoid the harmful sweets, fats, toxins, and chemical additives that trigger dietary imbalances.

THE GOAL POST THEORY OF
NUTRITIONAL BALANCE

These strict guidelines from above are the goal posts for establishing the strength of your balanced maintenance diet. And, there is total room for being yourself. No one single diet, food for food, sprout for sprout, can be followed by all people to insure a balanced optimal maintenance program. You see, your diet is as personal and as individualized as you are unique. With your interest in listening to the messages of your mind and body, you can tailor the guidelines of the Del Mar Maintenance Diet to satisfy your individual moods, and needs. Individual food tastes, nutritional sensitivities, and metabolic efficiencies vary as widely as do complexion, sex drive, skin color, hair styles, appearance, and body build.

Dietary habits invariably differ from individual to individual, from culture to culture, and from nation to nation. Why? Because your nutritional requirements for specific foods depend upon your body size, your physical activity, your work life, your sex life, your emotional health, your mental health, your spiritual progress, and your overall health status. Your environment, your climate, your cultural values, your social life, and your body efficiency also play a role. Naturally, these variables are subject to modification and change and, therefore, so is your diet.

A successful field goal means you score! By staying with the defined goal posts of your balanced maintenance diet, you can kick the field goal the way you feel best, see fit, and still score through the uprights.

Weight-loss diets, high-protein diets, low-protein diets, high-carbohydrate diets, low-carbohydrate diets, low-fat diets, and combinations thereof are popular. For defined periods of time, in very specific circumstances, they can serve a therapeutic purpose. Note that these above diets violate one or more of the criteria for a balanced Hi·Lite maintenance diet. Deviation from the right percentage of raw to cooked foods, alkaline to acid ratios, animal to vegetable proteins, or live to dead foods will not qualify any imbalanced diet as being able to, in spite of their claims, *maintain* optimal nourishment. The quality and right amount of natural fats and natural carbohydrates count. The Del Mar Maintenance Diet is the only truly balanced diet in print.

When you are following the Del Mar diet, all vital nutrients are present in the proper ratio and proportion. This bears the interest of well-being and fitness. THE ESSENCE OF THE DEL MAR NUTRITIONAL PROGRAM IS A WHOLESOME, LIVING, BALANCED DIETARY REGIMEN. The nutritional formula is to choose foods that are whole, that are abundant in vital life principles, and that combine together harmoniously to create an optimally balanced diet.

You, and only you, are responsible for carrying out your own nutritional policies. Make every meal an uplifting nutritional experience. The optimal diet keeps your mind alive, your spirit dazzling, and your body beautiful. It only comes to you from your own personal experience and self-awareness. It becomes your important responsibility to become fit in body, sound in mind, and filled with loving emotions. As you grow, develop, and change, you intelligently learn how to modify your optimal diet so it works for you. That is why the Del Mar Diet is actually an active on · going evolutionary process.

Experiencing nutritional wisdom is the purpose of this book. In consistently following the Del Mar diet, you experience the thrill of being *physically together*, *mentally clear*, and *whole-souled*. You know you have hit the stride of your optimal diet when you can sustain excellent health and prevent impending illness. When you can do whatever you want to do, for how ever long you want to do it, whatever it may be, whether it be in the ocean, on the jogging track, at work, in the bedroom, or on the dance floor, you are approaching the wholistic dimensions of optimal nourishment.

Hey, you, out there, I'm talking to you. One bright sunny day you may find yourself in the airways approaching Southern California. You may intercede on a conversation between the control tower and a ready-to-launch satellite.

"You have 21 days to land your craft. Cleanse to clear the runway. Detoxify for takeoff. Maintain to state your direction and course clearly. Fast to ground. Whip yourself into shape."

2: THE CLEANSING DIET:

Nutritional cleansing is a time-honored pearl of natural healing. The Cleansing Diet truly cleans out your system. The energized food nutrients in the Hi·Lite Cleansing Diet keep your metabolic machinery in unparalleled running order. This frees your tissues from collecting annoying grease and grime. You see, by eating the right combination of fresh wholesome living foods, your diet becomes a reliable self-regulating tool to purify your organs and your bodily fluids.

In the process of cleansing, poisons lodged in your vital organs are loosened up. The dead weight of devitalized toxins in bones, muscles, and joints are washed out. Your circulation gets a chance to fight off its internal debris. The Hi·Lite Cleansing Diet literally lightens you up as it lights up your cells.

HI·LITE NUTRITIONAL CLEANSING:
ALKALINE-ACID BALANCE

One thing for sure is that the Cleansing Diet makes for a focused adjustment in your body chemistry. The Hi·Lite Cleansing Diet is predominantly a hi-enzyme, raw, uncooked, highly alkaline, therapeutic diet. You see, an efficient live food cleansing diet is by definitio a hi-alkaline, walk-the-line diet. Abundant hi-enzyme, hi-lite raw foods such as sprouts, fresh fruits, raw vegetables, raw vegetable juices, and almonds create the highly alkaline residue of this diet. Nutritional overacidity is the most commonly misdiagnosed dietary disorder. In fact, overacidity is one of the earlier signs of impending degenerative toxemia.

One main objective of the Hi·Lite Cleansing Diet is to aid the kidneys in reestablishing the proper alkaline-acid balance of your overacidified body fluids. The result of internally bathing your cells in the biochemically healing waters of alkaline-acid balance buffers the acid poisons that build up from eating barrels of processed sweets, starches, and meats (and convenient nutritionless junk foods).

Before starting the diet consult the Physiology and Hi·Lights of Nutritional Cleansing.

PHYSIOLOGY OF THE 7·DAY NUTRITIONAL CLEANSING DIET

DAY 1	BREAK·INTO·IT	CUT INTO IT
DAY 2	BREAK·IT·UP	UPROOT THE TOXINS
DAY 3	BREAK·IT·DOWN	CLEAN IT OUT
DAY 4	BREAK·IT·LOOSE	EXCHANGE THE LIGHT FOR THE DARK
DAY 5	BREAK·IT·AWAY	PURIFY IT
DAY 6	BREAK·THROUGH·IT	BRIGHTEN IT UP
DAY 7	RENEW	CLEAR IT UP

The Cleansing Diet authentically solves the modern-day dilemma of what to do about the retention of environmental, nutritional, and emotional toxins, at a cellular level. This garbage is predominantly stored in the vital organs and the fat depots in your body.

DAY 1: BREAK · INTO · IT

The knife-like incision of Day 1 of the Hi·Lite Cleansing Diet cuts through the tissues and penetrates the membranes of your cellular walls. In this fashion, it *breaks· into* the minute spaces and cavities of structural poisons.

DAY 2: BREAK · IT · UP

On Day 2, the Hi·Lite Diet exposes the dark infestation of accumulated cellular toxic wastes. The hi·lite life-giving detergent action of hi-enzyme food *breaks· up* toxins that have accumulated in your cells.

DAY 3: BREAK · IT · DOWN

By Day 3, those fat depots and vital organs that are most toxic begin to be *broken· down* with the release of these poisons into your circulation.

DAY 4: BREAK·IT·LOOSE

The release of the poisons into the circulation *breaks·loose* a new *exchange* process. That is just the exchange we are looking for: replacing the old with the new. You see, the idea is to keep exchanging for good health. Every time you bring substantial quality into your body something of lesser quality that you have been holding onto osmotically leaves. In this way, you gradually *re·order* your system and restore proper alkaline-acid balance. Sickness leaves in exchange for health, malnourishment departs in exchange for nourishment, and you intelligently exchange negative poisons for real energy.

DAY 5: BREAK·IT·AWAY

In cutting it loose, the ongoing cellular release of murky foreign matter purifies your body fluids, while your blood gets refreshed, and the lymph becomes more clear. By Day 5 of the cleansing process, the internal purification has certainly taken hold. Genuine freedom from that which pollutes, impairs, and weakens is a simple unadulterated *break·away*.

DAY 6: BREAK·THROUGH·IT

Upward and onward to the positive excellence of a higher order is the sequential transparent *break·through*. Free of unneeded impurity, the body passes into a new level of wellness, liberated from stifling toxemic obstructions. Your thinking becomes loosened and straightforward, your emotions are unmistakable and unequivocal, and your body is serene. The calmness of your eternal love can be felt. The breakthrough can be seen in your new brightness. *Breaking·through·it* also helps you to clear out past regrets and disappointments.

DAY 7: RENEW

The nutritional arousal of your mental, physical, emotional, and spiritual purification is fundamental to activating your very own natural healing process. The effects are far-reaching. By Day 7 your cleansing exchange program creates a clear heart and *renews* the spirit.

Bear in mind that to initiate the healing effects of this hi-enzyme, alkaline, Hi·Lite Cleansing Diet it takes at least three days. During this entire 7-day plan your body learns to effectively handle its waste and eliminate its garbage. Usually by the third day, toxins begin to spill into your circulation and come into your consciousness. The symptoms of toxemia, fatigue, lethargy, irritability, headache, and a drugged dragged-out feeling correlate well with your pre-existing level of toxicity. Clearly, the cleaner your machine, the less you experience any discomfort in your cleansing program. In the beginning, to initiate your cosmic wellness program, and for the best results, it is essential that you stay on the Cleansing Diet for the seven full days and follow the directions carefully: to the exact prescription of the moment in time.

- **CUT INTO IT**
  - **UPROOT THE TOXINS**
    - **CLEAN IT OUT**
      - **EXCHANGE THE LIGHT FOR THE DARK**
        - **PURIFY IT**
          - **BRIGHTEN IT UP**
            - **CLEAR IT UP**

HI·LIGHTS OF NUTRITIONAL CLEANSING - I.
Blueprint For The Cleansing Diet

Early Morning	Good Morning! 15-20 minutes of aerobic exercise, deep breathing, and invigorating hydrotherapy, followed by:
Cosmic Interlude:	**THE CLEANSING BREAKFAST** (7:00-8:00 a.m.) (1) Fresh fruit juice in season (6 oz.) *15 minutes later:* (2) **HI · LITE FRUIT SALAD SUPREME** with 2-3 fresh seasonal fruits (1½ cups) and • 1-2 oz. almonds (approximately 15-25) • Nutritional supplements • Alfalfa sprouts (as many as you like)
Mid·morning	Herbal cleansing tea
Mid·day	Sunshine, relax your mind and body, followed by:
Cosmic Interlude:	**THE CLEANSING LUNCHEON** (12:30-2:00 p.m.) - with two options
Option A· **(for colder climates)**	(1) Fresh carrot juice (6 oz.) *15 minutes later:* (2) **A HI · LITE LEAFY·GREEN CHLOROPHYLL SALAD:** Raw sprouted garden-crisp vegetables with romaine lettuce, sprouts, tomato, and 3 select fresh, raw, green vegetables, with your choice of HERBAL SALAD DRESSING* and *one* of the following: • 2 tsp. sunflower or sesame seeds • 2 tsp. sesame-tahini butter on a crisp celery stalk • ½ avocado with or without salsa • 1-2 celery sticks with 1 Tbsp. crunchy peanut butter per stalk • Nutritional supplements
Option B· **(for warmer climates)**	(1) Fresh fruit juice in season (6 oz.) *15 minutes later:* (2) **CLEANSING FRUIT AND NUT SALAD** with 2-3 oz. mixed nuts, including almonds • alfalfa sprouts (as many as you like) • Nutritional supplements
Mid·afternoon	Herbal cleansing tea
Evening	15 minutes of relaxation and / or meditation, followed by:
Cosmic Interlude:	**THE CLEANSING VEGETARIAN DINNER** (5:30-7:00 p.m.) (1) Fresh carrot, carrot-celery, or carrot-celery-beet juice (8 oz.) *15 minutes later:* (2) **SPROUTED GARDEN·FRESH SALAD** with a variety of fresh, raw vegetables and • 2 tsp. sunflower seeds added to salad (3) STEAMED GREEN VEGETABLE COMBINATION (a platter of 2-3 steamed green vegetables) · or BROCCOLI-MIXED GREENS VEGETABLE SOUP (I bowl) (4) STARCHY CARBOHYDRATE, to be chosen from: • Baked potato, I medium (no butter or salt) • corn on the cob, 1 ear (no butter or salt) • Baked yam, I medium • Steamed or baked squash, 1 medium Note: Use CLEANSING CHILI SALSA or avocado to flavor your starches. Omit sunflower seeds when using avocado on starches. • Nutritional supplements
After Dinner	Herbal cleansing tea

*This applies to your dinner salad as well. See recipes.

Guidelines For The Cleansing Diet
Foods Allowed On The Hi·Lite Cleansing Diet

Seasonal Fresh Fruits and Fruit Juices	yes	All fresh fruits in season. Avoid sweetened, frozen, canned, packaged fruits. No dried fruits. The bottom line is one **HI·LITE FRESH FRUIT SALAD SUPREME** per day. Emphasize lemons, pink grapefruit, grapes, berries, mangos, strawberries, watermelon.
Fresh Vegetables and Raw Vegetable Juices	yes	All fresh vegetables with an emphasis on raw leafy greens and steamed broccoli, zucchini, and string beans. Avoid frozen, canned, wilted, salted, oiled vegetables. Avoid white head lettuce.
Sprouts	yes	Living sprouts are essential to the Cleansing Diet. Emphasize alfalfa, bean, and sunflower seed sprouts.
Nuts	yes	Almonds are an alkaline staple to the morning Cleansing Diet. Walnuts, cashews, and brazil nuts are acceptable along with almonds for your mixed nuts at lunch. Avoid peanuts. Avoid salted, oiled, commercially roasted nuts. Raw or home roasted nuts are acceptable.
Nut Butter	yes	Unhydrogenated, unsalted peanut or almond butter is highly nutritious on a crisp celery stalk. Avoid all other nut butters. Nut butters can be raw or home roasted.
Seeds	yes	Raw or home roasted sunflower seeds and sesame seeds are the seeds of choice for the Cleansing Diet. Eat your seeds with green vegetables and not with fruits.
Natural Starchy Carbohydrates	yes	Baked potatoes, corn on the cob, yams, steamed or baked squash (acorn, winter, spaghetti squash) without butter, oil, or salt is a staple of the Cleansing Dinner.
Beverages	yes	Corresponding seasonal fruit juice twice daily. Carrot, carrot-celery, or carrot-celery-beet juice twice a day.
Herbs	yes	Peppermint, Rose Hips, Lemon Grass, Hibiscus Flower are good cleansing herbs made into herbal tea.
Seasonings	yes	Avoid coffee, soft and diet drinks, alcohol. Avoid all sugar and salt. Red cayenne pepper, fresh garlic, fresh onion, apple cider vinegar, and lemon are special all-purpose cleansing condiments.
Whole Grains	no	
Legumes	no	
Dairy Products	no	
Eggs	no	
Flesh Foods	no	

The bottom line is:
- 1 fruit salad with at least 1 oz. almonds for breakfast.
- 1 vegetable salad at dinner.
- 1 starchy carbohydrate at dinner.
- 2 glasses raw vegetable juice daily.
- 2 glasses seasonal fruit juice daily.

HI·LIGHTS OF NUTRITIONAL CLEANSING - III.
Food Groupings For The Cleansing Diet

When the proper food ingredients on the Cleansing Diet are combined together appropriately on the basis of sound food-combining, you come up with seven fundamental food groups on the Cleansing Diet.

GROUP 1:   **HI·LITE FRUIT SALAD SUPREMES**

Fruits have seasons of peak nutritional value. Eat only the fresh fruits in season. The Hi·Lite Fruit Salad Supreme of choice changes with the seasons.

Spring:
- (1) **SOUTH AMERICAN TROPICAL FRUIT SALAD** (papaya, pineapple, banana)
- (2) **ZESTY SPRING SALAD** (pineapple, banana, strawberry)
- (3) **CHERRY SUPREME SALAD** (cherry, peach, banana)
- (4) **GRAPE DELIGHT SALAD** (green, purple, and red grapes)
- (5) **MANGO DAYBREAK DELIGHT** (mango, pineapple, banana)

Summer:
- (1) **SUMMER MELON SALAD** (cantelope, watermelon, papaya)
- (2) **CANTALOUPE MELON SALAD** (cantaloupe, watermelon, banana)
- (3) **APRICOT SUNSHINE SALAD** (apricot, peach, and plum, cherry, or grape)
- (4) **HAWAIIAN FRUIT SALAD** (papaya, mango, pineapple)
- (5) **SOUTH AMERICAN TROPICAL FRUIT SALAD** (papaya, pineapple, banana)
- (6) **RADIANT BERRY SALAD** (berries, peach, apricot)
- (7) **MANGO PEACH SALAD** (mango, peach, banana)
- (8) **CHERRY, FRIAR PLUM SALAD** (cherries, Friar plum, nectarine, or other variety of plum)
- (9) **NECTARINE PEACH SALAD** (nectarine, peach, cherries)
- (10) **SUMMER GRAPE SALAD** (grapes, cherries, banana)

Autumn:
- (1) **MIXED APPLE SALAD** (Pippin apple, MacIntosh apple, Golden Delicious apple)
- (2) **WALDORF APPLE SALAD AMBROSIA** (Pippin apple, pear, banana)
- (3) **AUTUMN ENERGY SALAD** (banana, papaya, Pippin apple)
- (4) **PEACEFUL PEAR SALAD** (pear, papaya, banana)
- (5) **GRAPE CURE SALAD** (green grape, red grape, or any mono grape, and lots of them)
- (6) **MIXED PEAR SALAD** (Bartlett, D'Anjou, and Bosc pears)
- (7) **EARLY AUTUMN SALAD** (Cantaloupe with banana or grapes)

Winter:
- (1) **SOUTH AMERICAN TROPICAL FRUIT SALAD** (pineapple, papaya, banana)
- (2) **WINTER CITRUS SALAD** (orange, pineapple, pink grapefruit)
- (3) **ORANGE WONDERLAND SALAD** (orange, pineapple, banana)
- (4) **PINK GRAPEFRUIT WINTER SALAD** (pink grapefruit, orange, banana)
- (5) **PAPAYA PARADISE SALAD** (orange, papaya, banana)

GROUP 1a: **FRESH FRUIT JUICES**

Spring:
Fresh orange juice
Fresh grapefruit juice
Fresh pineapple juice
Fresh papaya juice
Fresh papaya-pineapple juice

Summer:
Watermelon juice
Cantaloupe juice
Papaya juice

Autumn:
Fresh apple juice
Fresh pineapple juice
Fresh pear juice
Fresh orange juice

Winter:
Fresh orange juice
Fresh grapefruit juice
Fresh pineapple juice

GROUP 2:   MELTZER HI·LITE LEAFY·GREEN CHLOROPHYLL SALADS

(1) **SPROUTED GARDEN-FRESH DINNER SALAD** (romaine lettuce, tomato, sprouts, parsley, red onion, red cabbage, carrot)

(2) **GARDEN-GREEN CHLOROPHYLL SALAD** (romaine lettuce, spinach, Swiss chard, parsley, sprouts, tomato, carrot)

(3) **SPICE-OF-LIFE SPINACH SALAD** (spinach leaves, romaine lettuce, sprouts, tomato, red onion, celery)

(4) **COOL CUCUMBER SALAD** (cucumber, carrot, green bell pepper, radishes, romaine lettuce, sprouts, tomato)

(5) **MEXICAN CABBAGE SALAD** (red cabbage, green cabbage, red onion or green onion, romaine lettuce, tomato)

(6) **AVOCADO-TOMATO GRANDE SALAD** (avocado, tomato, romaine lettuce, sprouts, cucumber, beet)

(7) **RADIANT RADISH SALAD** (radishes, red onion, romaine lettuce, sprouts, tomato, parsley)

(8) **RAW MUSHROOM SALAD** (mushrooms, romaine lettuce, sprouts, tomato, cucumber, celery)

(9) **CAULIFLOWER SALAD** (cauliflower, celery, mushrooms, romaine lettuce, sprouts, tomato)

(10) **GARDEN PEA SALAD** (Chinese snow peas, green peas, green or red bell pepper, romaine lettuce, sprouts, tomato)

(11) **JICAMA-BEET TREAT** (jicama, beet, carrot, romaine lettuce, sprouts, tomato)

(12) **MUSTARD GREENS SALAD** (mustard greens, beet greens, dandelion greens, sprouts, tomato)

(13) **SUPER SPROUTS SALAD** (mung bean sprouts, alfalfa sprouts, sunflower seed sprouts, romaine lettuce, tomato)

(14) **CUCUMBER-BEET SALAD** (cucumber, beet, red onion, romaine lettuce, sprouts, tomato)

(15) **BASIC AVOCADO SALAD** (avocado, beet, beet greens, red onion, romaine lettuce, sprouts, tomato)

(16) **VEGETABLES-FROM-THE-SEA SALAD** (romaine lettuce, avocado, celery, tomato, sprouts, kelp, dulse, or nori)

GROUP 2a: FRESH VEGETABLE JUICES

(1) Fresh carrot juice
(2) Fresh carrot-celery juice
(3) Fresh carrot-celery-beet juice
(4) Fresh carrot-celery-beet-parsley juice
(5) Fresh carrot-celery-beet-cucumber juice
(6) Fresh carrot-celery-parsley juice
(7) Fresh carrot-celery-stringbean juice

GROUP 3:   STEAMED GREEN VEGETABLE COMBINATIONS

(1) **BROCCOLI-ZUCCHINI VEGETABLE PLATTER** (broccoli, zucchini, string beans)

(2) **ASPARAGUS-BROCCOLI MEDLEY** (asparagus, broccoli, zucchini)

(3) **CAULIFLOWER MIXED VEGETABLE PLATTER** (cauliflower, zucchini, broccoli)

(4) **BRUSSELS SPROUT MIXED VEGETABLE PLATTER** (Brussels sprouts, zucchini, green bell peppers)

(5) **GREEN BEAN VEGETABLE COMBINATION** (green beans, carrots, spinach or chard)

(6) **CHINESE STEAMED VEGETABLE COMBINATION** (Chinese snow peas, bok choy, jicama, carrots)

(7) **STEAMED CARROT-PEAS VEGETABLE PLATTER** (green peas, carrots, broccoli)

(8) **BROCCOLI-MIXED GREENS VEGETABLE SOUP** (broccoli, zucchini, string beans or combinations of the above)

GROUP 4:   NATURAL STARCHY CARBOHYDRATES

(1) Baked potato

(2) Corn on the cob

(3) Baked yams

(4) Baked squash

GROUP 5:   CLEANSING DIET VEGETABLE PROTEIN SPECIALTIES

(1) ½ avocado

(2) 2 tsp. sunflower or sesame seeds

(3) 1 Tbsp. sesame-tahini butter stuffed into crisp celery stick

(4) 1 Tbsp. crunchy peanut butter stuffed into crisp celery stick

(5) 1 Tbsp. almond butter stuffed into crisp celery stick

GROUP 6:   MIXED NUT PROTEIN COMBINATIONS

(1) 1 oz. almonds — 1-2 oz. cashews

(2) 1 oz. almonds — 1-2 oz. walnuts

(3) 1 oz. almonds — 1-2 oz. brazil nuts

GROUP 7:   HERBAL SALAD DRESSINGS

(1) **LEMON-GARLIC DRESSING** (juice of a lemon, cloves, garlic, oregano, kelp)

(2) **VINAIGRETTE DRESSING** (apple cider vinegar, garlic, lemon, kelp, oregano, paprika)

(3) **ITALIAN HERBAL DRESSING** (tomatoes, apple cider vinegar, garlic, onion, dill, paprika)

(4) **AVOCADO GREEN DRESSING** (avocado, lemon, garlic, cayenne). Use this dressing as a substitute for sunflower or sesame seeds on a basic Meltzer Chlorophyll Afternoon Luncheon Salad.

(5) **"MELTZER CHILI SAUCE"** (tomato, green peppers, oregano, red cayenne pepper, green onions, fresh chili, or chili powder)

(6) **KELP-FROM-THE-SEA DRESSING** (kelp, garlic, onion, red cayenne, chili, apple cider vinegar, ginger root)

(7) **DYNAMIC HERBAL DRESSING** (lemon, scallions, parsley, celery seed, paprika, basil, oregano, rosemary)

HI · LIGHTS OF NUTRITIONAL CLEANSING — IV.
GOLDEN RULES FOR CLEANSING

Cleansing has some fundamental rules to guide you to select and combine your food properly. Follow these simple rules and you will be rewarded mentally and physically.

RULE NO. 1:
- EAT THREE MEALS A DAY.

RULE NO. 2:
- BREAKFAST BETWEEN 7:00 to 8:00 a.m. FOR 30 MINUTES.
- Drink 1 glass of **fresh fruit juice** from the corresponding season in **Group 1a** (6 oz.). 15 minutes later:
- Select 1 **FRUIT SALAD SUPREME** from **Group 1** in accordance with the appropriate season.
- Add 1-2 ounces almonds to your fruit salad.
- Alfalfa sprouts are optional.

RULE NO. 3:
- LUNCH BETWEEN 12:30 to 2:00 FOR 30 MINUTES.
- Drink 1 glass **fresh vegetable juice** from **Group 2a** (6 oz.).
- Select 1 **LEAFY-GREEN CHLOROPHYLL SALAD** from **Group 2**.
- Select 1 **VEGETABLE PROTEIN SPECIALTY** from **Group 5.**
- Select 1 **HERBAL SALAD DRESSING** from **Group 7**.

OR

- Drink 1 glass of **fresh fruit juice** from the corresponding season in **Group 1a** (6 oz.). 15 minutes later:
- Select 1 **FRUIT SALAD SUPREME** from **Group 1** in accordance with the appropriate season.
- Select 1 **MIXED NUT PROTEIN COMBINATION** from **Group 6**.

RULE NO. 4:
- DINE BETWEEN 5:30 and 7:00 p.m. allow at least 30 minutes and up to 90 minutes for a pleasant, enjoyable dinner.
- Drink 1 glass of **fresh vegetable juice** from **Group 2a** (8 oz.).
- Select 1 **LEAFY-GREEN CHLOROPHYLL SALAD** from **Group 2**.
- Add 2 tsp.sunflower seeds to the salad.
- Choose 1 **HERBAL SALAD DRESSING** from **Group 7.**
- Select 1 **STEAMED GREEN VEGETABLE COMBINATION** from **Group 3.**
- Choose 1 **NATURAL STARCHY CARBOHYDRATE** from **Group 4.**

RULE NO. 5:
- AVOID SNACKING.

RULE NO. 6:
- AVOID BREAD, GRAINS, LEGUMES, DAIRY, OR FLESH PROTEINS.

RULE NO. 7:
- TAKE 30 MINUTES AT LEAST TO ENJOY EACH MEAL.

RULE NO. 8:
- BE CERTAIN TO DRINK 6-8 GLASSES OF FLUID EACH DAY.
- BETWEEN MEALS DRINK ONLY HERBAL TEAS. Camomile, comfrey and peppermint are noted for their cleansing properties.

RULE NO. 9:
- SEASON YOUR FOODS WITH THE CLEANSING HERBS OF GARLIC, RED CAYENNE PEPPER, AND FRESH RED CHILI. LEMON AND LIME JUICE, APPLE CIDER VINEGAR, AND ONIONS COMPLETE THE 7 BASIC CONDIMENTS TO THE CLEANSING DIET.

THE LOW-PROTEIN VEGETARIAN DIET

The Hi·Lite Cleansing Diet is a low-protein, low-fat, high in simple natural carbohydrate diet. It provides anywhere from 15-25 grams of complete protein, depending upon how many nuts and how much nut butter you eat. Cleansing diets are purposely low-protein.

A low-protein vegetarian diet is most conducive to a gentle housecleaning. The short-term low-protein Cleansing Diet arouses the subtle inner vibrations of your sparkling, vital life energies. And the Hi·Lite Cleansing Diet conserves metabolic energy normally utilized to digest and metabolize protein.

You see, the power behind this extra energy now becomes a vital reservoir. First it is shunted into electrifying the cleansing. Then the autopurification process of the liver is stimulated, and the pancreas is given a low-profile vacation because it needs to digest less protein. In fact, depending on your health, you can survive and do very well on raw juices, fruits, and live raw food without very much protein for as long as 2-3 weeks at a time. This, of course, depends on your overall nutritional status as well as the strength of your mind, body, and spirit. And seven days of cleansing is usually all that is necessary to cleanse at any one time. Remember that a cleansing diet is not intended to be a maintenance plan.

Yes, you are getting enough protein on the Cleansing Diet. All but those who are malnourished or in the very lower nightshade of the "twilight zone" can afford to forgo their high protein habit and receive the benefits of the low-protein Hi·Lite Cleansing Diet. What is the twilight zone? Well, before you can fully appreciate what I mean, there is something you ought to know about your level of well-being.

DR. MELTZER'S HEALTH STAIRCASE:
Size Up Your Level of Wellness

THERE ARE FIVE FUNDAMENTAL CATEGORIES OF HEALTH STATUS:

I. Optimal Nourishment: Optimal Wellness

II. Suboptimal Nourishment: Partial Wellness

III. Mediocre Nourishment: Average Health

IV. Poor Nourishment: Poor Health

V. Malnourishment: Symptomatic Dis-ease

These categories correspond to the five levels of *nutritional* status as protrayed on the following graph:

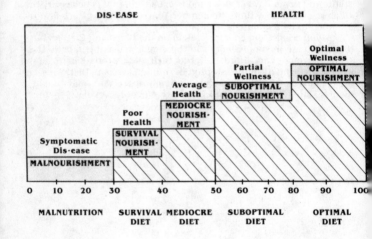

The 21-Day Del Mar Diet

Looking directly at the chart the 100 point is the best of health and the zero is the death point. Fifty is the cut-off point between wellness to the right and illness to the left. At the top of the stairs is Category I (C·I), *Optimal Nourishment*. O·N is characterized by:

- **Real HAPPINESS.**
- **Consistent SEXUAL FUL-FILLMENT and satisfaction.**
- **Daily PEACE OF MIND.**
- **A self-reliant, POSITIVE MENTAL ATTITUDE.**
- **The absence of any physical or mental symptoms of illness.**
- **A joyful sense of WELL-BEING in a time of stress or crisis.**

- **A strong, PHYSICALLY FIT BODY.**
- **Lasting EMOTIONAL FULFILLMENT.**
- **IDEAL BODY WEIGHT.**
- **The joy of SPIRITUAL PROSPERITY.**
- **Ongoing EMOTIONAL STABILITY.**
- **MEANINGFUL RELATIONSHIPS.**
- **BALANCED LIFESTYLE.**
- **NUTRITIONAL BIOCHEMICAL BALANCE.**

Your optimal diet is high-level nutritional wellness. It is the nutritional domain of optimal wellness. It is also a firm prerequisite to optimal nourishment. Only through your optimal diet can the *dynamic* state of experiencing real and total *nutritional balance* be realized. It is not a fixed point on the curve. Optimal diet has depth, movement, and is capable of evolutionary growth and development. In fact, your optimal diet is the catalyst to the total nourishment of your whole being. You feel terrific and you look great.

All the way on the other side of the staircase is C·V, *Malnourishment*. It is characterized by a dis-eased body, a sick mind, and an ailing spirit. This is the inferior level of health status where your chronic bodily complaints of living can be verified by a conventional medical physical examination.

When you get down to operating at 30 percent or less of your optimal level of functioning, you have the symptoms of serious disease. *MALNOURISHMENT* is a nutrient-deficient state. Malnutrition is a frank, *quantitative* nutritional deficiency state. Quantitative malnutrition results from the *under*-consumption of substantial life-supporting food nutrients.

ARE YOU IN THE TWILIGHT ZONE?

C·II, III, and IV, *Suboptimal, Mediocre,* and *Poor Nourishment,* respectively, make up the "Twilight Zone." The twilight zone is a state of confusion and disorder. By definition, it is a state of imbalance. The twilight zone is the dimly illuminated fog of less than total wellness. There are various shades of gray to describe this imperfect clarity. You can be in the hazy mist of the upper twilight zone or stuck in the inner darkness of the lower twilight zone. In either case, you are floating in the *Ether*. That is, your mind, body, and emotions are anesthetized to total wellness.

C·IV, *Poor Nourishment*, means that you are in a survival consciousness. To Robert, a 34-year-old married car salesman, living was having a job and just getting by. He existed from one crisis in his life to the next. He was a survivor. Robert went through life saying, "What happened?" He was content to barely outlast the threats and damage from the self-created storms in his environment.

Survival consciousness is characterized by poor random habits of eating, living, and drinking for the sake of existence or security. You are inconsistent at best. Depression is hard to shake. In fact, you are existing and not living. When you are immersed in survival, you see life as a struggle to get by. When a pick-pocket sees a saint, all he sees are his pockets.

Survival nutrition is the direct result of being poorly nourished.

The *survival diet* means exactly that. You are eating to exist and existing to eat. Your diet just gets you through each day. Your nutri-

C·III, *Mediocre Nourishment*, is the ordinary middle-of-the-road middle-quality health status. The great majority of people are in this particular catagory. Mediocre nourishment correlates well with average health of not really being well. Your energy level is inconsistent. Sometimes you have it, and lots of times you don't. You are living at best up to only 50% of your full potential. And surviving. Sometimes you are up, and often you are down. You look o.k., and that's better than you feel. Your mind and body are in a state of dynamic disequilibrium between positive health factors and the self-destructive forces of illness. You are nourished well enough to be free of any signs of illness. On the other hand, you are sufficiently overstressed and undernourished that you are unable to ward off slow-to-appear, long-standing maladies. That is why the creeping crud of mediocre nourishment is called the category of Non-symptomatic Disease.

Nutritional mediocrity is also very commonplace. A mediocre diet signifies that you are getting some of the right nutrients and plenty of the wrong nutrients. Assimilation is out-of-order. Actually, mediocre nutrition is just one stage above survival nutrition. Both, however, are on a collision course to body breakdown.

C·II, *Suboptimal Nourishment*, speaks for suboptimal wellness. You are by no means sick, and usually feel pretty good, but at the same time, you are not feeling great, or looking great, or overflowing with endless energy and happiness. This is why Suboptimal Nourishment is also called Subclinical Wellness. It is a state of partial wellness. It commonly categorizes the scores of well-wishing health seekers. They intuitively know there is more vigor and substance to life. And there is a wide chasm between their experience and the full limits of their potential.

The suboptimal diet describes usually good food selections that need to be a bit more balanced and consistent. Often, eating habits and food combinations are faulty. Assimilation is incomplete, and your body chemistry is not fully balanced. Nutritional cleansing and nutritional detoxification are inadequate.

NUTRITIONAL TWILIGHT ZONE

The great silent majority of our fellow citizens, whether they are willing to admit it or not, are walking around in the vulnerable twilight zone of nutritional imbalance. And this is understandable. How can you possibly *know* what you haven't ever experienced? Sally, after six years of marriage with David, didn't realize she wasn't having a full orgasm until she slept with Steven. It wasn't until Larry cut out the junk food from his diet that he discovered what it was like to wake up in the morning feeling good. When Betty stopped automatically reaching for her late-afternoon cocktail, she began to feel undrugged and had glimpses of being alive when the sun went down.

It is human nature for individuals to settle into what they are doing and often unnecessarily accept what they are used to as being the best life has to offer. Our modern day merry-go-round lifestyle gets us nowhere and becomes a worrisome routine. It is common to be caught up on this kind of treadmill. It is easy to lose perspective when you are on the periphery of healthy living. You can think you're healthy, but until you experience optimal nourishment, you will never know what you're missing.

Can you identify yourself below among the variety of symptoms that tell you that you are a victim of the nutritional twilight zone?

The symptoms of this nutritional twilight zone include the following. Check yourself out.

BODILY DYSFUNCTION

_____ Fatigue

_____ Lethargy

_____ Obesity

_____ Physical illness

_____ Sexual frustration

_____ Headache

_____ Insomnia

_____ Indigestion

_____ Back troubles

_____ Constipation

_____ Menstrual disorders

_____ Poor appetite

_____ Low energy levels

EMOTIONAL DYSFUNCTION

_____ Depression

_____ Emotional unfulfillment

_____ Constant emotional crises

_____ Fluctuating emotional states

_____ Buried fears

_____ Retained hostilities

_____ Chronic guilt

_____ Repressed anger

_____ Emotional inconsistency

_____ Chronic frustrations

_____ Emotional numbness ("not enough love in your heart")

_____ Disabling insecurities

MENTAL DYSFUNCTION

_____ Anxiety

_____ Confusion

_____ High stress levels

_____ Inability to relax

_____ Poor time management

_____ Laziness

_____ Negative thinking

_____ Poor self-esteem

SPIRITUAL DYSFUNCTION

_____ Purposelessness

_____ Imbalanced lifestyle

_____ Low enthusiasm

_____ Joylessness

Your optimal diet, the Hi·Lite nutritional program, is a valued therapeutic cornerstone for treating *all* of these above symptoms.

It is often recommended to spend one week getting yourself clear about your personal living habits—your eating, sleeping, mental, emotional, and working habits. The following chart will facilitate the process. To get the most out of your 21 Hi·Lite days to wellness, it is of the utmost importance to have a feeling of who you are and what you need to change. And, until you make the time to keep track of yourself, you won't know.

SELF-ASSESSMENT

Remember, your first active step can very well be to give yourself a full week to get to know yourself better. On the following charts sketch out your relationship with your eating habits and how you choose to spend the 24 hours in each of the next seven days.

Chart No. I gives you the opportunity to write down everything you eat for one whole week. It also gives you an overview of your current lifestyle. Chart No. II is for keeping a record of the location of your meals and what you are doing while you eat. In Chart No. III the timing of your meals, your mood, and degree of hunger each time you eat can also be recorded. With this newfound self-correcting consciousness of how your eating habits affect your lifestyle, you will be ripe for the new you to surface in the ensuing 21 days to radiant well-being.

CHART NO. I.
Dietary And Activity Record

	MONDAY	TUESDAY	WEDNESDAY	THURSDAY	FRIDAY	SATURDAY	SUNDAY
Morning Breakfast							
Moods							
Thoughts							
Snacks							
Activities							
Afternoon Lunch							
Moods							
Thoughts							
Snacks							
Activities							
Evening Dinner							
Moods							
Thoughts							
Snacks							
Activities							
Hours Slept							
Wake-up Time							
Sex							

Weekly Summary of Moods, Thoughts, Feelings, Stresses and Activities:

The 21-Day Del Mar Diet

CHART NO. II
Eating Habits Survey

Each time you eat a meal, darken in a triangle ◣ Each time you snack mark an X in the triangle ◺ᵡ
Mark appropriate location. Score in adjacent triangle from 1-8 what you are doing during the meal or snack. * (See Below)

PLACE	DAY 1	DAY 2	DAY 3	DAY 4	DAY 5	DAY 6	DAY 7
HOME - Dinner table or other designated eating place							
T.V. ROOM							
KITCHEN - Not at table							
BEDROOM							
OFFICE							
CAR							
RUSHING out the door							
RESTAURANT							
FRIEND'S HOME designated eating place							
JUNK FOOD STAND							
WORK AREA							
OTHER							

1. Only eating
2. Reading Paper, Book, Letter
3. Watching T.V. or listening to Radio
4. Paying Bills
5. Studying
6. Working
7. Cooking
8. Telephone
9. Other

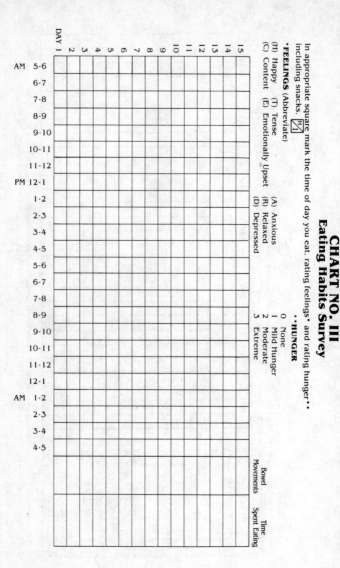

CHART NO. III
Eating Habits Survey

In appropriate square mark the time of day you eat, rating feelings* and rating hunger** including snacks. ☑

* **FEELINGS** (Abbreviate)

(H) Happy   (T) Tense   (A) Anxious
(C) Content   (E) Emotionally Upset   (R) Relaxed
     (D) Depressed

** **HUNGER**

0   None
1   Mild Hunger
2   Moderate
3   Extreme

DAY	1	2	3	4	5	6	7	8	9	10	11	12	13	14	15
AM 5-6															
6-7															
7-8															
8-9															
9-10															
10-11															
11-12															
PM 12-1															
1-2															
2-3															
3-4															
4-5															
5-6															
6-7															
7-8															
8-9															
9-10															
10-11															
11-12															
12-1															
AM 1-2															
2-3															
3-4															
4-5															
Bowel Movements															
Time Spent Eating															

In summary, the "twilight zone" is a relative state of nutritional deficiency. This ether of dietary imbalance results from consuming nutrient-poor devitalized, processed, unnatural food. Excess meat, sugar, oil, milk, dairy, salt, starch, and refined carbohydrates are poisonous to your body. This imbalance is aggravated by inferior eating habits. Keep in mind that the twilight zone of nutritional imbalance is caused by varying degrees of:

- *Overconsumption of bad food.*
- *Underconsumption of high-quality nutritional fuel.*
- *Destructive irregular eating habits.*
- *Improper food combinations.*
- *Overconsumption of good food.*

High levels of stress, disorderly lifestyles, negative mental attitudes, destructive emotional habits, and lack of emotional nourishment create further imbalance in your mind, body, and spirit by interfering with the assimilation of proper nutrients.

Unless you are frankly malnourished, you may think you are well-nourished. Stop kidding yourself. Peace is not the absence of war. Health is not the absence of disease. Optimal nutrition is not the absence of malnutrition. People associate wellness with not being sick. When they don't have to see the doctor they figure they must be well. That kind of thinking needs to be changed. Survival nutrition, mediocre nutrition, and suboptimal nutrition are *all* varying kinds of modern-day malnutrition. They are, in reality, *qualitative* states of malnutrition. You are overloaded in destructive nutrients.

TIME FOR A CHANGE

Everyone living in the above twilight zone is wise to make significant dietary changes. In fact, were I to tell you that unless you made fundamental changes in your nutritional lifestyle you would get deathly ill, everybody who believes me and really cares about his life, and I mean *everybody*, would be willing to take the time and be ready to make the changes immediately. Start with one week of Nutritional Cleansing. Then be sure to follow-up with one week of Nutritional Detoxification, and then one week of Nutritional Maintenance.

THE BALANCING OF YOUR BODY CHEMISTRY FROM YOUR HI·LITE DIETARY PROGRAM IS THE STEPPING STONE TO OPTIMAL NOURISHMENT.

It is irrational to expect your mind, body, and spirit to reach the most natural peak experiences without the defined benefit of optimal nutrition. How can you possibly expect your life to be balanced when your body chemistry is not?

GETTING CLEAR GETS YOU OUT OF
THE TWILIGHT ZONE

Richard was suffering with the "poor-man syndrome." He was not rich in spirit, companionship, love, time, or health. He was in the twilight zone.

Richard was a successful, well-educated, 37-year-old banker. He was extremely frustrated. The night before he came to see me he was celebrating his anniversary at a downtown restaurant. Of all the nights to pick up some food poisoning! I prescribed a potassium-rich, alkaline, green vegetable broth. He responded quickly. One week later he returned to my clinic with a sore throat and a high fever. That made two infections in two weeks. He wanted to know what was going on.

"Dr. Barney, I feel like I'm falling apart. My body is breaking down and my mind is scattered. I have always been successful. Right now I just can't keep it together. I have had two complete company physicals in the last month. They tell me there is nothing wrong with me. And that I should have my head examined. I still feel weak and tired and I can't shake a cold. I know there's something that's not right. I don't feel like myself anymore. What's wrong with me, Doc?"

I told Richard that he would need to take a comprehensive look at himself as a whole person. I scheduled him for a more thorough work-up.

Richard had always been hard-driving and aggressive. Ever since he could remember he had found it nearly impossible to relax. He couldn't let go. His mid-day energy level was low and falling. By the end of a working day he was wiped out.

He was well-dressed and very professional looking. To look at him, you'd think he was as happy as a lark. He had an establishment job, a beautiful home in the suburbs, a handsome silver '59 Porsche, and an ocean-view office. All this was topped off with a large staff.

He spent little time at anything outside his high-pressured job. His wife was threatening divorce. He was busy and absorbed in his work. With rising interest rates, Richard was becoming more and more pessimistic about his financial future. Over the past three years he had become progressively more obsessed with his business responsibilities. His relationship with his wife became technical and functional. He often refused to communicate patiently. He did not want to discuss personal matters. They began to live in different parts of the house. Richard spent his weekends playing with the kids and his weeknights sleeping on the couch. He usually fell asleep in front of the TV. His wife was wiped out and would go to sleep alone. Their conversation had become short and tense. Richard started keeping to himself.

He became more and more depressed. He found himself working harder and having less fun in his life. About this time he began to feel

HI·LIGHTS OF NUTRITIONAL CLEANSING · I.
Blueprint For The Cleansing Diet

Early Morning	Good Morning! 15-20 minutes of aerobic exercise, deep breathing, and invigorating hydrotherapy, followed by:
Cosmic Interlude:	**THE CLEANSING BREAKFAST** (7:00-8:00 a.m.) (1) Fresh fruit juice in season (6 oz.) *15 minutes later:* (2) **HI · LITE FRUIT SALAD SUPREME** with 2-3 fresh seasonal fruits (1½ cups) and • 1-2 oz. almonds (approximately 15-25) • Nutritional supplements • Alfalfa sprouts (as many as you like)
Mid·morning	Herbal cleansing tea

Mid·day	Sunshine, relax your mind and body, followed by:
Cosmic Interlude:	**THE CLEANSING LUNCHEON** (12:30-2:00 p.m.) - with two options
Option A· (for colder climates)	(1) Fresh carrot juice (6 oz.) *15 minutes later:* (2) **A HI · LITE LEAFY·GREEN CHLOROPHYLL SALAD:** Raw sprouted garden-crisp vegetables with romaine lettuce, sprouts, tomato, and 3 select fresh, raw, green vegetables, with your choice of HERBAL SALAD DRESSING* and *one* of the following: • 2 tsp. sunflower or sesame seeds • 2 tsp. sesame-tahini butter on a crisp celery stalk • ½ avocado with or without salsa • 1-2 celery sticks with 1 Tbsp. crunchy peanut butter per stalk • Nutritional supplements
Option B· (for warmer climates)	(1) Fresh fruit juice in season (6 oz.) *15 minutes later:* (2) **CLEANSING FRUIT AND NUT SALAD** with 2-3 oz. mixed nuts, including almonds • alfalfa sprouts (as many as you like) • Nutritional supplements
Mid·afternoon	Herbal cleansing tea

Evening	15 minutes of relaxation and/or meditation, followed by:
Cosmic Interlude:	**THE CLEANSING VEGETARIAN DINNER** (5:30-7:00 p.m.) (1) Fresh carrot, carrot-celery, or carrot-celery-beet juice (8 oz.) *15 minutes later:* (2) **SPROUTED GARDEN·FRESH SALAD** with a variety of fresh, raw vegetables and • 2 tsp. sunflower seeds added to salad (3) STEAMED GREEN VEGETABLE COMBINATION (a platter of 2-3 steamed green vegetables) - or BROCCOLI-MIXED GREENS VEGETABLE SOUP (l bowl) (4) STARCHY CARBOHYDRATE, to be chosen from: • Baked potato, 1 medium (no butter or salt) • corn on the cob, 1 ear (no butter or salt) • Baked yam, 1 medium • Steamed or baked squash, 1 medium Note: Use CLEANSING CHILI SALSA or avocado to flavor your starches. Omit sunflower seeds when using avocado on starches. • Nutritional supplements
After Dinner	Herbal cleansing tea

*This applies to your dinner salad as well. See recipes.

HI· LIGHTS OF NUTRITIONAL CLEANSING · II

Guidelines For The Cleansing Diet
Foods Allowed On The Hi · Lite Cleansing Diet

Seasonal Fresh Fruits and Fruit Juices	yes	All fresh fruits in season. Avoid sweetened, frozen, canned, packaged fruits. No dried fruits. The bottom line is one **HI·LITE FRESH FRUIT SALAD SUPREME** per day. Emphasize lemons, pink grapefruit, grapes, berries, mangos, strawberries, watermelon.
Fresh Vegetables and Raw Vegetable Juices	yes	All fresh vegetables with an emphasis on raw leafy greens and steamed broccoli, zucchini, and string beans. Avoid frozen, canned, wilted, salted, oiled vegetables. Avoid white head lettuce.
Sprouts	yes	Living sprouts are essential to the Cleansing Diet. Emphasize alfalfa, bean, and sunflower seed sprouts.
Nuts	yes	Almonds are an alkaline staple to the morning Cleansing Diet. Walnuts, cashews, and brazil nuts are acceptable along with almonds for your mixed nuts at lunch. Avoid peanuts. Avoid salted, oiled, commercially roasted nuts. Raw or home roasted nuts are acceptable.
Nut Butter	yes	Unhydrogenated, unsalted peanut or almond butter is highly nutritious on a crisp celery stalk. Avoid all other nut butters. Nut butters can be raw or home roasted.
Seeds	yes	Raw or home roasted sunflower seeds and sesame seeds are the seeds of choice for the Cleansing Diet. Eat your seeds with green vegetables and not with fruits.
Natural Starchy Carbohydrates	yes	Baked potatoes, corn on the cob, yams, steamed or baked squash (acorn, winter, spaghetti squash) without butter, oil, or salt is a staple of the Cleansing Dinner.
Beverages	yes	Corresponding seasonal fruit juice twice daily. Carrot, carrot-celery, or carrot-celery-beet juice twice a day.
Herbs	yes	Peppermint, Rose Hips, Lemon Grass, Hibiscus Flower are good cleansing herbs made into herbal tea.
Seasonings	yes	Avoid coffee, soft and diet drinks, alcohol. Avoid all sugar and salt. Red cayenne pepper, fresh garlic, fresh onion, apple cider vinegar, and lemon are special all-purpose cleansing condiments.
Whole Grains	no	
Legumes	no	
Dairy Products	no	
Eggs	no	
Flesh Foods	no	

The bottom line is:
- 1 fruit salad with at least 1 oz. almonds for breakfast.
- 1 vegetable salad at dinner.
- 1 starchy carbohydrate at dinner.
- 2 glasses raw vegetable juice daily.
- 2 glasses seasonal fruit juice daily.

HI·LIGHTS OF NUTRITIONAL CLEANSING - III.
Food Groupings For The Cleansing Diet

When the proper food ingredients on the Cleansing Diet are combined together appropriately on the basis of sound food-combining, you come up with seven fundamental food groups on the Cleansing Diet.

GROUP 1:   HI·LITE FRUIT SALAD SUPREMES

Fruits have seasons of peak nutritional value. Eat only the fresh fruits in season. The Hi·Lite Fruit Salad Supreme of choice changes with the seasons.

Spring:
(1) **SOUTH AMERICAN TROPICAL FRUIT SALAD** (papaya, pineapple, banana)
(2) **ZESTY SPRING SALAD** (pineapple, banana, strawberry)
(3) **CHERRY SUPREME SALAD** (cherry, peach, banana)
(4) **GRAPE DELIGHT SALAD** (green, purple, and red grapes)
(5) **MANGO DAYBREAK DELIGHT** (mango, pineapple, banana)

Summer:
(1) **SUMMER MELON SALAD** (cantelope, watermelon, papaya)
(2) **CANTALOUPE MELON SALAD** (cantaloupe, watermelon, banana)
(3) **APRICOT SUNSHINE SALAD** (apricot, peach, and plum, cherry, or grape)
(4) **HAWAIIAN FRUIT SALAD** (papaya, mango, pineapple)
(5) **SOUTH AMERICAN TROPICAL FRUIT SALAD** (papaya, pineapple, banana)
(6) **RADIANT BERRY SALAD** (berries, peach, apricot)
(7) **MANGO PEACH SALAD** (mango, peach, banana)
(8) **CHERRY, FRIAR PLUM SALAD** (cherries, Friar plum, nectarine, or other variety of plum)
(9) **NECTARINE PEACH SALAD** (nectarine, peach, cherries)
(10) **SUMMER GRAPE SALAD** (grapes, cherries, banana)

Autumn:
(1) **MIXED APPLE SALAD** (Pippin apple, MacIntosh apple, Golden Delicious apple)
(2) **WALDORF APPLE SALAD AMBROSIA** (Pippin apple, pear, banana)
(3) **AUTUMN ENERGY SALAD** (banana, papaya, Pippin apple)
(4) **PEACEFUL PEAR SALAD** (pear, papaya, banana)
(5) **GRAPE CURE SALAD** (green grape, red grape, or any mono grape, and lots of them)
(6) **MIXED PEAR SALAD** (Bartlett, D'Anjou, and Bosc pears)
(7) **EARLY AUTUMN SALAD** (Cantaloupe with banana or grapes)

Winter:
(1) **SOUTH AMERICAN TROPICAL FRUIT SALAD** (pineapple, papaya, banana)
(2) **WINTER CITRUS SALAD** (orange, pineapple, pink grapefruit)
(3) **ORANGE WONDERLAND SALAD** (orange, pineapple, banana)
(4) **PINK GRAPEFRUIT WINTER SALAD** (pink grapefruit, orange, banana)
(5) **PAPAYA PARADISE SALAD** (orange, papaya, banana)

GROUP 1a: FRESH FRUIT JUICES

Spring:		Summer:	
Fresh orange juice		Watermelon juice	
Fresh grapefruit juice		Cantaloupe juice	
Fresh pineapple juice		Papaya juice	
Fresh papaya juice			
Fresh papaya-pineapple juice			

Autumn:		Winter:	
Fresh apple juice		Fresh orange juice	
Fresh pineapple juice		Fresh grapefruit juice	
Fresh pear juice		Fresh pineapple juice	
Fresh orange juice			

GROUP 2:   MELTZER HI·LITE LEAFY·GREEN CHLOROPHYLL SALADS

(1) **SPROUTED GARDEN·FRESH DINNER SALAD** (romaine lettuce, tomato, sprouts, parsley, red onion, red cabbage, carrot)

(2) **GARDEN·GREEN CHLOROPHYLL SALAD** (romaine lettuce, spinach, Swiss chard, parsley, sprouts, tomato, carrot)

(3) **SPICE·OF·LIFE SPINACH SALAD** (spinach leaves, romaine lettuce, sprouts, tomato, red onion, celery)

(4) **COOL CUCUMBER SALAD** (cucumber, carrot, green bell pepper, radishes, romaine lettuce, sprouts, tomato)

(5) **MEXICAN CABBAGE SALAD** (red cabbage, green cabbage, red onion or green onion, romaine lettuce, tomato)

(6) **AVOCADO·TOMATO GRANDE SALAD** (avocado, tomato, romaine lettuce, sprouts, cucumber, beet)

(7) **RADIANT RADISH SALAD** (radishes, red onion, romaine lettuce, sprouts, tomato, parsley)

(8) **RAW MUSHROOM SALAD** (mushrooms, romaine lettuce, sprouts, tomato, cucumber, celery)

(9) **CAULIFLOWER SALAD** (cauliflower, celery, mushrooms, romaine lettuce, sprouts, tomato)

(10) **GARDEN PEA SALAD** (Chinese snow peas, green peas, green or red bell pepper, romaine lettuce, sprouts, tomato)

(11) **JICAMA·BEET TREAT** (jicama, beet, carrot, romaine lettuce, sprouts, tomato)

(12) **MUSTARD GREENS SALAD** (mustard greens, beet greens, dandelion greens, sprouts, tomato)

(13) **SUPER SPROUTS SALAD** (mung bean sprouts, alfalfa sprouts, sunflower seed sprouts, romaine lettuce, tomato)

(14) **CUCUMBER·BEET SALAD** (cucumber, beet, red onion, romaine lettuce, sprouts, tomato)

(15) **BASIC AVOCADO SALAD** (avocado, beet, beet greens, red onion, romaine lettuce, sprouts, tomato)

(16) **VEGETABLES·FROM·THE·SEA SALAD** (romaine lettuce, avocado, celery, tomato, sprouts, kelp, dulse, or nori)

GROUP 2a: FRESH VEGETABLE JUICES

(1) Fresh carrot juice
(2) Fresh carrot-celery juice
(3) Fresh carrot-celery-beet juice
(4) Fresh carrot-celery-beet-parsley juice
(5) Fresh carrot-celery-beet-cucumber juice
(6) Fresh carrot-celery-parsley juice
(7) Fresh carrot-celery-stringbean juice

DAY 4: BREAK·IT·LOOSE

The release of the poisons into the circulation *breaks·loose* a new *exchange* process. That is just the exchange we are looking for: replacing the old with the new. You see, the idea is to keep exchanging for good health. Every time you bring substantial quality into your body something of lesser quality that you have been holding onto osmotically leaves. In this way, you gradually *re·order* your system and restore proper alkaline-acid balance. Sickness leaves in exchange for health, malnourishment departs in exchange for nourishment, and you intelligently exchange negative poisons for real energy.

DAY 5: BREAK·IT·AWAY

In cutting it loose, the ongoing cellular release of murky foreign matter purifies your body fluids, while your blood gets refreshed, and the lymph becomes more clear. By Day 5 of the cleansing process, the internal purification has certainly taken hold. Genuine freedom from that which pollutes, impairs, and weakens is a simple unadulterated *break·away*.

DAY 6: BREAK·THROUGH·IT

Upward and onward to the positive excellence of a higher order is the sequential transparent *break·through*. Free of unneeded impurity, the body passes into a new level of wellness, liberated from stifling toxemic obstructions. Your thinking becomes loosened and straightforward, your emotions are unmistakable and unequivocal, and your body is serene. The calmness of your eternal love can be felt. The breakthrough can be seen in your new brightness. *Breaking·through·it* also helps you to clear out past regrets and disappointments.

DAY 7: RENEW

The nutritional arousal of your mental, physical, emotional, and spiritual purification is fundamental to activating your very own natural healing process. The effects are far-reaching. By Day 7 your cleansing exchange program creates a clear heart and *renews* the spirit.

Bear in mind that to initiate the healing effects of this hi-enzyme, alkaline, Hi·Lite Cleansing Diet it takes at least three days. During this entire 7-day plan your body learns to effectively handle its waste and eliminate its garbage. Usually by the third day, toxins begin to spill into your circulation and come into your consciousness. The symptoms of toxemia, fatigue, lethargy, irritability, headache, and a drugged dragged-out feeling correlate well with your pre-existing level of toxicity. Clearly, the cleaner your machine, the less you experience any discomfort in your cleansing program. In the beginning, to initiate your cosmic wellness program, and for the best results, it is essential that you stay on the Cleansing Diet for the seven full days and follow the directions carefully: to the exact prescription of the moment in time.

- **CUT INTO IT**
  - **UPROOT THE TOXINS**
    - **CLEAN IT OUT**
      - **EXCHANGE THE LIGHT FOR THE DARK**
    - **PURIFY IT**
      - **BRIGHTEN IT UP**
        - **CLEAR IT UP**

MEATS: AVOID MEAT PROTEIN. Red meat is loaded with synthetic chemicals. Meat is a toxic fuel that fills you up artificially and gives you a drugged hyped-up energy level. Beef protein is obstructive. It hurts your pancreas. Red meat protein consumption results in heavy accumulation of acid residue toxins in the body. This damages nerves and especially joints. Meat has been cited as a risk factor to the increased incidence in rectal and colon cancer. Over-Proteinzation, or eating more animal protein than you need, whether it be meat, fish, or chicken, is a negative cultural phenomenon.

FATS: High fat levels clog the circulation. They are major contributory risk factors for hardening of the arteries, diabetes, and obesity. Excess fat in your diet increase your vulnerability to breast cancer, cancer of the uterus, as well as gall bladder cancer and other malignancies. Too much meat or dairy is a common nutritional turn-over. Animal fats, in particular meat and lard are high in cholesterol. They have a molesting influence on your hormonal balance. Grease prematurely rusts your system.

REFINED CARBOHYDRATES: White rice impairs your liver's ability to be the detoxifying machine that it can be. Avoid sweets, and artificially sweetened foods.

SOFT DRINKS: A cultural rip-off, nutritionally. They contain hidden caffeine, sugar, and artificial chemicals.

MILK: The most exaggerated food in the world for adults and teen-agers. Milk is very mucus forming. Pasteurized milk overstimulates the upper respiratory passages, ears, nose, throat, sinuses, and the lungs to oversecrete. Pasteurized milk allergies are common. Digestive gland function and assimilation is also compromised from excessive mucus formation.

CAFFEINE: Caffeinism is a social ritual. Overstimulation to the nerves, adrenals, and heart is hazardous to your well-being. Headaches and breast lumps are common.

You are smart to avoid the excess of any nutrient that increases your risk to suffer with a diet-related deficiency. Why do I make such a fuss over these frequently-advertised easy access food items? Because they have a corrosive effect on the integrity of your digestive enzymes. The net effect of this pernicious influence is incomplete assimilation of vital life-giving nutrients.

With the help of your optimal diet, your body will learn to assimilate your food well. This means that your mind opens, body solidifies, emotions prosper, and spirit reaches out. It also suggests that you get what you need from what you choose to eat. Your optimal diet is a very powerful form of preventive medicine. When your optimal diet is well assimilated, you can completely satisfy the appetites of your whole body.

Eating your way to wellness is an orderly, natural process. It naturally evolves from responsible nutritional decision making.

Nevertheless, adolescent teenagers and many on-the-go employees often fall victim to eating what is convenient . . . plenty of sweets, fats, soft drinks, delicatessen meats, chemically processed acid-forming beef, fried chicken, and shellfish. Or, you start missing meals because you are rushed. On-the-go nutrition results in nutritional imbalance because of inferior assimilation of minerals, vitamins, and vegetable proteins. Avoid the harmful sweets, fats, toxins, and chemical additives that trigger dietary imbalances.

THE GOAL POST THEORY OF NUTRITIONAL BALANCE

These strict guidelines from above are the goal posts for establishing the strength of your balanced maintenance diet. And, there is total room for being yourself. No one single diet, food for food, sprout for sprout, can be followed by all people to insure a balanced optimal maintenance program. You see, your diet is as personal and as individualized as you are unique. With your interest in listening to the messages of your mind and body, you can tailor the guidelines of the Del Mar Maintenance Diet to satisfy your individual moods, and needs. Individual food tastes, nutritional sensitivities, and metabolic efficiencies vary as widely as do complexion, sex drive, skin color, hair styles, appearance, and body build.

Dietary habits invariably differ from individual to individual, from culture to culture, and from nation to nation. Why? Because your nutritional requirements for specific foods depend upon your body size, your physical activity, your work life, your sex life, your emotional health, your mental health, your spiritual progress, and your overall health status. Your environment, your climate, your cultural values, your social life, and your body efficiency also play a role. Naturally, these variables are subject to modification and change and, therefore, so is your diet.

A successful field goal means you score! By staying with the defined goal posts of your balanced maintenance diet, you can kick the field goal the way you feel best, see fit, and still score through the uprights.

Weight-loss diets, high-protein diets, low-protein diets, high-carbohydrate diets, low-carbohydrate diets, low-fat diets, and combinations thereof are popular. For defined periods of time, in very specific circumstances, they can serve a therapeutic purpose. Note that these above diets violate one or more of the criteria for a balanced Hi·Lite maintenance diet. Deviation from the right percentage of raw to cooked foods, alkaline to acid ratios, animal to vegetable proteins, or live to dead foods will not qualify any imbalanced diet as being able to, in spite of their claims, *maintain*

TAKE CONTROL TO GET THE POWER

The natural hi-enzyme diets of Hi·Lite Cleansing, Detoxification, Maintenance, and juice fasting, working in harmony with the seasonal changes is your optimal diet. By adhering to the natural rhythm of quarterly cleansing and mid-seasonal detoxification you assume ground control power and gain control of your life. It is the unique food combinations and timing of this Del Mar diet that gives you the power to:

- *Cleanse* destructive toxins from the blood and the lymph to enhance the healing powers of the circulation.

- *Purify* the mind and emotions. Costly impurities from the central nervous system and the ductless glands are removed in exchange for a positive mental attitude and inner happiness. This allows for your positive feelings and emotions to flow without the obstructions of a toxic bodily physiology.

- *Detoxify* poisoned and overworked vital organs, such as liver, kidneys, and intestines, and make room for positive life-giving nutrients.

- *Activate* the body's natural detoxifying powers to render noxious wastes and poisons harmless.

- *Eliminate* harmful sediment, plaque, wastes, deposits, and toxins from the body.

- *Arrest* uncalled for bodily decay and degeneration.

- *Restore* nourishment to worn out nerves and exhausted glands.

- *Revitalize* the sex glands.

- *Rejuvenate* the spirit.

- *Elevate* your consciousness.

- *Create* optimal super · nutrition.

- *Maintain* optimal nourishment.

- *Sustain* optimal nourishment.

RHYTHMIC BLUEPRINT FOR YOUR SEASONAL DEL MAR DIET

SPRING EQUINOX — March 20°			**SUMMER EQUINOX — June 20°**		
	3/20-4/30	Maintenance Diet — juice fast 1 day a week		6/20-7/31	Maintenance Diet — juice fast 1 day a week
MID-SEASONAL DETOXIFI-CATION	5/1-5/5	Detoxification Diet	**MID-SEASONAL DETOXIFI-CATION**	8/1-8/5	Detoxification Diet
	5/6-6/9	Maintenance Diet — juice fast 1 day a week		8/6-9/9	Maintenance Diet — juice fast 1 day a week
SEASONAL CLEANSING	6/10-6/15	Cleansing Diet	**SEASONAL CLEANSING**	9/10-9/15	Cleansing Diet
	6/16-6/19	Maintenance Diet		9/16-9/19	Maintenance Diet
AUTUMNAL EQUINOX — Sept. 20°			**WINTER EQUINOX — December 20°**		
	9/20-10/31	Maintenance Diet — juice fast 1 day a week		12/20-1/31	Maintenance Diet — juice fast 1 day a week
MID-SEASONAL DETOXIFI-CATION	11/1-11/5	Detoxification Diet	**MID-SEASONAL DETOXIFI-CATION**	2/1-2/5	Detoxification Diet
	11/6-12/9	Maintenance Diet — juice fast 1 day a week		2/6-3/9	Maintenance Diet — juice fast 1 day a week
SEASONAL CLEANSING	12/10-12/15	Cleansing Diet	**SEASONAL CLEANSING**	3/10-3/15	Cleansing Diet
	12/16-12/19	Maintenance Diet		3/16-3/19	Maintenance Diet

You can do the first 21 Days whenever you want. And then keep up the beat. In Light of your quarterly cleansing, it is best to begin the basic 21 Day Plan right at the start, or at the middle of a new season.

Once you have completed the initial 21 Days, plug into the natural rhythm of the diet. In effect, then, the Del Mar Diet is based upon the fundamentals principle of preventative medicine: keep yourself balanced to stay well. In harmony with yourself, you stand the most favorable chance to keep in harmony with your changing environment. The truth is that when you are well nourished you can stay in charge of *your* life. Your optimal diet gives you the adaptability to stay internally balanced with the changing forces in the world around you.

WHAT HAPPENS AFTER 21 DAYS?

Thanks for asking. There is something more you need to know about the Del Mar Diet. The balance of nature is its teacher.

To be well and stay that way you have to keep in balance with the natural changes in the climate and weather in your environment. Nature is always changing. And so are you. A great deal of your health has to do with keeping abreast with the natural changes taking place as the seasons change. When you do it right, it is called being in tune with nature.

Optimal health is actually the ability to stay well in spite of the inevitable changes in the weather. Have you ever noticed how most everyone at work or at school is coming down with a "what's going around virus" at the very time there is a change in the season. That is where the term "under the weather" comes from. It is the responsibility of your optimal diet to sustain your natural rhythm so you're not thrown off course. Who can afford the loss of time from work or play?

THE RHYTHM METHOD OF THE DEL MAR DIET

The rhyme and reason of the Del Mar Diet is to keep you centered. The focus is to stay in balance with the seasonal changes. To do this the Del Mar Diet is a quarterly plan based on the four seasons. Within each season the balance and nutritional support rotates around the timing of your Cleansing, Detox, Maintenance and Juice Fasting Plan.

SEASONAL TIMING COUNTS

The prescription of the Del Mar nutritional program looks like this. Within each 90 day period you follow:

1. **A BALANCED MAINTENANCE DIET** for approximately 75-85% of the time.

2. **CLEANSING, DETOXIFICATION, OR FASTING DIETS** are the nutritional therapy of choice for approximately 15-25% of the days.

The frequency and duration of the Del Mar Cleansing, Detoxification, and Fasting protocols are prescribed to keep you leveled off and equalized.

I. AT EACH EQUINOX:
Practice 5 days on the *Del Mar Cleansing Diet.* It is best to begin 10 days before each seasonal change (equinox). The seasonal cleansings are as follows:

- Spring seasonal cleansing 7-10 days before March 20-22 (mark your calendar on March 10)

- Summer seasonal cleansing 7-10 days before June 20-22 (mark your calendar on June 10)

- Autumn seasonal cleansing 7-10 days before September 20-22 (mark your calendar on September 10)

- Winter seasonal cleansing 7-10 days before December 20-22 (mark your calendar on December 10)

II. AT THE MIDSEASON:
Practice 5 days on the *Del Mar Detoxification Diet.* Start at the *midway point* between the seasonal changes. Therefore, the mid-seasonal detoxification is as follows:

- Spring mid-seasonal detoxification the first week in May.
- Summer mid-seasonal detoxification the first week in August.
- Autumn mid-seasonal detoxification the first week in November.
- Winter mid-seasonal detoxification the first week in February.

III. JUICE FAST 1 DAY A WEEK:
Choose the first working day of each week to juice it. After 2 years on the Del Mar Diet juice fasting can be substituted for the cleansing and detoxification diets at the seasonal and mid-seasonal junctures. Then, cleanse and detoxify for 5 days respectively after your seasonal and mid-seasonal juice fasting.

STRIKE A BALANCE

On purpose, your optimal diet balances out your body chemistry. It brings you into internal balance. In sticking to the proper food combinations the Del Mar diet brings you into harmony with your emotional and physiological needs. Your body gets trim and strong and your moods get stabilized. Your spirit comes alive and your mental attitude shines in the Light.

The balance in the Del Mar Diet keeps the engines of your mind churning. It provides an abundant reservoir of energy so you can function very well. The exceptional quality of the Del Mar Diet also feeds your emotional and spiritual wellness.

How you begin to feel is the magic of the program. Balancing the chemistry in your cells and bodily fluids turns on your very own orderly enzymatic vital life energies. As you Lighten up, your whole being comes alive! In turn, this leads to greater **Strength** and further **Balance**.

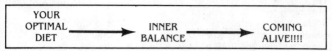

YOUR OPTIMAL DIET ⟶ INNER BALANCE ⟶ COMING ALIVE!!!!

THE DEL MAR DIET WORKS!
KEEP TO THE RHYTHM

What naturally follows when you eat right is that you experience, maybe for the first time in your adult life, the sensational thrill of being fully alive. How is it that one diet can get you balanced and further keep you that way? The secret lies in the **rhythm method** of the Del Mar Diet. The program is actually a series of diets. The complete Del Mar Diet is made up of a Cleansing, Detoxification, and Maintenance Diet. A juice fasting program is also part of your Detoxification routine.

Your search for the right diet is over. Knowing how and when to cleanse, detoxify, juice fast or maintain is what keeps you well. This is all you have to know.

- **The Cleansing Diet:** To cleanse your body, clarify your mind, brighten up your spirit, and get rid of the accumulated poisons of modern day living.
- **The Detoxification Diet:** To strengthen your immune system and purge your body of deep-seated poisons.
- **The Maintenance Diet:** To nourish your whole being to wellness.
- **The Fasting Program:** To keep your metabolism rejuvenated and your weight under control.

The lifetime, *"Keep-it-Off"* Del Mar Permanent weight loss program is a variation on the above theme. Knowing how and when to Cleanse, Detoxify and Juice Fast makes it easy to maintain your ideal weight.

HOW TO USE THE PROGRAM

The basic 21 Day Del Mar Diet is divided into three weeks.

WEEK 1: *Nutritional Cleansing:* to lighten up your life

WEEK 2: *Nutritional Detoxification:* to purge out bodily poisons

WEEK 3: *Nutritional Maintenance:* to balance out your body chemistry

The Del Mar Diet is for everyone. Teenagers, adults, and senior citizens can all do very well. Children under 14 and pregnant women only need the Maintenance Plan.

Those of you in good health, looking for optimal health, are rewarded by sticking to the 21 day plan. Invariably you feel terrific. For most, you lose 7-10 pounds in the first two weeks. By the end of three weeks you shed 10-15 pounds. You see, the Maintenance Diet levels you off, and keeps it off. Depending upon how much you exercise, you can sometimes lose 20 pounds or more. In any event, wellness and not just losing unsightly pounds is the focus for your program.

It is very interesting that as you break down the poisons, folks in mediocre health may experience some fatigue or vague symptoms of withdrawal. This usually goes away by the end of the Cleansing Diet or shortly after you begin week two Detox. See the risks of the Cleansing Diet page 15 for details. Individuals in poor health, or those who suffer with functional hypoglycemia, diabetes, cancer and other metabolic disturbances can follow the 21 Day Del Mar Diet with a few modest modifications. In these cases, it is well advised that you be under the supervision of your family doctor.

For those of you that need to lose more than 15 pounds, you have a weight problem. Do something about it. Begin with the easy to follow, "Rapid, 21 day" weight loss segment of the program. "See Chapter 8, page 143." It is very close to the original 21 Day Del Mar Diet. It differs because it has more juice fasting, and follows through with a Take · Charge · Keep · Slim Maintenance Diet.

THE COMPLETE
21-Day
Del Mar Diet

beginning of the consumer movement towards questioning our standard nutritional values. Every time the word 'balanced' was mentioned, it brought down the house with applause.

After the fifteenth time the speaker mentioned the term 'balanced diet,' I can vividly remember what transpired. I started to feel a bit uneasy. My pulse quickened. I thought to myself either I was the dumbest person in the whole convention hall, or I'm the only one to have the guts to ask. I respectfully stood up. I raised my hand. My words reverberated throughout the El Cortez Hotel. "Mr. Speaker, I beg your pardon. My name is Barnet G. Meltzer. I am a surgical resident at the University of California. Please enlighten me. *What exactly do you mean by a balanced diet?*"

"A balanced diet is, you know, well, er, it's usually umm, let's see, hmm, I think, you know, er, it's usually, well let's see, maybe. . . . Everybody knows what a balanced diet is . . . ah . . . um . . . a balanced diet is . . . ahh. . . ." Well, after much humming and hawing, the speaker came right to the point. "*A balanced diet is a balanced diet.*" After a short discussion, I realized that there was much confusion. There was absolutely no consensus as to what were the ingredients of a balanced diet.

I looked to that evening's lecture as one of the turning points in my life. That night I strengthened my resolve and made up my mind to determine exactly what constitutes a balanced diet. I spent the next 12 years learning the secrets of man's optimal diet. And what I found out was so drastically different than what I was led to believe. I have never been the same. It was incredible. I have treated thousands of patients in my office in Southern California. I did a nutritional research tour of Mexico and Central America. I spent nearly three years on horseback riding through the wilds of the South American Andes studying the diets of very sheltered, primitive peoples. I returned to my beloved California. There was no doubt about it.

MAN'S OPTIMAL DIET IS RICH IN:

- **Fresh fruits.**
- **Fresh raw vegetables.**
- **The vegetable proteins of staple whole grains and legumes.**

Big business, TV commercials, restaurants, magazine and newspaper food features encourage the consumption of dangerous toxic devitalized foods. I witnessed the No. 1 nutritional deficiency in South America to be *under*consumption malnutrition. I realized that *over*consumption malnutrition was truly the No. 1 nutritional deficiency in the United States. It was the direct result of overeating poor-quality preservative-rich foods.

This suicidal nutritional condition is intimately related to the menancing level of inertia and mediocrity threatening our very lifestyles. Simply take a look at your level of stress, your degree of sexual satisfaction, your level of emotional fulfillment or happiness, or your blood pressure, your triglyceride level, your cholesterol, or your weight to know what long-term effects your present dietary lifestyle has created. You are what you choose to eat. Your relationship with your diet has the same meaningful connection as does the ripened fruit growing from a healthy tree. Let me put the cards on the table, you can play them, or request a new deal.

rundown. He dragged at work. He was getting more and more tired.

His sex life had completely deteriorated. "I don't think my relationship with my wife is going to last. Before, the future looked bright and rosy. Now I'm not so sure. I don't have the energy to keep on top of my business or my *nature* any longer."

Everything in his life was changing. His mind, his body, his home life, and his sex life were all on the verge of collapse. Richard didn't quite know how to cope with his situation. He felt trapped. He was surely vulnerable. He was becoming more and more pessimistic about his one success — his career. "If only I had more time and more money, I'm sure I could get it together."

Of great concern to me were his living habits. He used alcohol, caffeine, tobacco, and sugar for a "pick-me-up" during the day. He loved coffee and sweetened donuts. He was a typical "sugar freak." He habitually put three to four teaspoons of table sugar in each cup of coffee. In the afternoon he treated himself to chocolate-chip ice cream or a chocolate milkshake. His after-dinner reward was snacking on his favorite candy bar. He was fed up with the advice he was getting from the family doctor who could find nothing organically wrong with him.

THE CAUSE: IMBALANCED LIVING

Although complete examinations by other physicians found nothing wrong with Richard, *he did not get to first base with me.* My preventive medicine evaluation revealed that his relationships and his body chemistry were severely imbalanced. His nerves were shot. He was suffering from being overworked, undernurtured, and nutritionally abused. "I suspect that you have low blood sugar. My secretary is going to schedule you for a five-hour glucose-tolerance blood test." The test results left no question about it. Sure enough, Richard's fatigue, low energy level, and poor resistance were due to a *Reactive Hypoglycemic,* or low blood sugar, condition. Incidentally, some 85 percent of all people are walking around with this condition.

When I reviewed his medical profile with him, I made it abundantly clear that he was losing in the most important areas of his life. He was not happy. He was physically out of shape. His mind was negative. His emotions were depressed. His spirit was low. He was not in control of his life.

"You see, Richard, you are walking around in the fog of the twilight zone. Richard, health and disease are at opposite ends of the rainbow." I handed Richard Dr. Barney's diagram which subdivides your level of health into five categories.

"You are not alone, Richard. The great majority of individuals fall into Category II, III or Category IV. They are either tiptoeing in the twilight zone of ready-to-strike potential illness or are experiencing sub-optimal wellness.

"When you were thoroughly examined by your physicians, they determined that you did not have any Category V serious illness. That is why they told you that nothing was wrong with you. The great majority of people who feel something is wrong are usually right about themselves. It's just that *conventional medicine can only detect advanced illness*. It can't diagnose potential weakness. You can check out completely well on the physical exam and laboratory tests—and still be on the tightrope. At point 34 or 35 on the staircase, you're on your course to becoming a disease statistic.

"You can see clearly that health isn't really the absence of disease. *It is the realization of the whole person.*

"Rich, your being here tells me that you want to get well. You have been living inside of a self-destructive shell. Your soul is suffocating. Your emotions need more than a breath of fresh air. Your mind is a victim of your own pessimistic, negative thinking. You have thrown your whole life out of balance. Your poor energy level is a warning sign from your body. It is time to set yourself in motion. You are ready to move out of the twilight zone of potential disaster. With genuine determination, you can overcome your difficulties and move into a *state of wellness*. With the Meltzer Diet and the Meltzer Wellness Program you will learn to *BECOME STRONG AND BALANCED IN MIND, BODY, EMOTION, AND SPIRIT*. This will create internal balance. When you are in harmony with yourself, you will then be in the most favorable position to be in harmony with your environment.

"In this world there are few things for sure. Do you realize that change is one of the only constants in your life? Even at this moment, everything is different. *Life is always changing. The secret to being on top of your mind and body is how you flow with these changes.* Believe me, Richard, through it all you can stay in balance. With this wellness program I am going to outline for you, you will be capable of keeping it all together."

Under my supervision, Richard initiated the "21 Days to Wellness" program. Right away he changed his attitude. He began to think positively. He took charge of his life. With this prescription for wellness he squared away his emotional stress:

EXERCISE: 1. A regular daily yogic-aerobic fitness program: Richard began jogging for 20 minutes each day before breakfast. He practiced some hatha yoga and stretching exercises for 10 minutes before lunch and then again before dinner.

LIFESTYLE: 2. Creating a balance: He re-evaluated and changed his priorities. He found out he could make the time for himself and his family.

RELAXATION: 3. A stress-management, stress-reduction program:
In following the Meltzer Wellness Program he took the active responsibility for his life. By establishing healthful habits he eliminated 85% of his previous disorderly, unpredicable, circumstantial, emotional stress. He became the actor instead of the reactor. He learned how to let it all go.

DIET: 4. "21 Days to Wellness Dietary Regime":
After completing the 3-week dietary program, he continued with a high fiber, high complex carbohydrate, low fat, moderate protein (55 grms.) diet. Richard eliminated heavy fats, meats, sweets, coffee, cigarettes, alcohol, and chemical preservatives from his diet. The timely ingestion of specialized vegetable protein at mid-morning and mid-afternoon helped to overcome his metabolic low blood sugar.

Richard soon began to feel better. His morning workouts became one of the regular high points of his day. He got totally involved in his natural, hi-enzyme, balanced, vegetarian based, high-fiber, low-cholesterol, low-fat diet. He got so enthusiastic with his program that, after a busy day at work, he would often come home and prepare the meal for his family.

At the end of one year, Richard looked his age. Previously, he had looked seven years older. He was relaxed, happy, and productive. He was enjoying his life for the first time.

I asked Richard what his thoughts were about the year that had just gone by.

"I now feel healthy. I see within myself a marked change for the better. I see that I can actually control my health. This is very exciting for me. This year I have elimated sugar, coffee, meat, and cigarettes!

"I still need to have more discipline in my daily routine. I especially need to get down on myself in the areas of meditation, exercise, and getting out of bed. But, I am learning to be a positive thinker. My increased enthusiasm has made life a new challenge for me. I am getting more out of my work, my personal life, and whole loving relationships.

"To be able to wake up each morning with a positive feeling and go to bed each night with a sense of accomplishment is indeed a blessing!"

Richard had taken responsibility for becoming his own health expert. He had taken over. He brought his life together. He got it together with his wife and kids. He beat his low blood sugar condition. He was able to put his emotional stress into perspective. He became optimistic about his job. Before the year was over, he was promoted to manage a new branch office of his bank. He had come to terms with his realities. As an added bonus to becoming healthy, he realized that his life, indeed, was very rich.

IN TUNE WITH LIFE

Optimal nourishment (O·N) is the freedom to come together dynamically with change. Your level of health is measured by your ability to keep in balance with the movement of your life. The winds of change can be mild or overpowering. They can rattle your heart, strain your pocketbook, and tax the limits of your mind.

Meet up to the challenges in your life with a consistency that defies the imagination. This consistency calls into play all the details of physical, mental, emotional, and spiritual health.

In a nutshell, O·N enables you *to endure the psychic pain going on in your life*. You can turn any conflict into a growth-oriented experience.

Isn't it interesting that everybody's life has some daily frustrations. Uncertainties are a real part of life and living. Wherever there is life, you will find challenges and hurdles. No matter who you are or what your circumstances, you create your own life. You have to make your own waves or the waves make you.

FINE TUNING IS IN ORDER

Be wise. Review your daily habits. "21 Days to Wellness" will help you make the necessary adjustments now. Stay cool and calm. Courage is built upon converting small or large threatening experiences into moral triumphs. Right now, simply get in touch.

You can learn to deal successfully with whatever comes your way.

• *Be ready at all times.*

• *Deal positively with whatever is happening in your life.*

OPTIMAL HEALTH IS THE ABILITY TO THRUST FORWARD AND OVERCOME YOUR OBSTACLES.

You can learn to spiritually jump the high hurdles.

Let's go back to the very beginning. Your diet is the nucleus of your upcoming transformation. It is your practical initiation into life as it really is.

LOSE 3·7 POUNDS IN ONE WEEK

In studying the nutritional tables, you can see that the Hi·Lite Cleansing Diet is essentially an 800-1200 calorie diet, averaging some 16-20 grams of complete protein. This makes it a moderately low-caloric and efficient weight loss diet. Keep in mind that *a calorie is a calorie is a calorie.* For those who prefer not to lose weight, it is important to eat more food and often double up proportionally on the size of your portions to more easily approach a 2,000+ calorie diet. For example, eating an extra bowl of fresh fruit can be as much as 200-250 calories. Substantial amounts of natural starches (baked potato, corn-on-the-cob), nut butters, and fruits usually will maintain your weight. By strictly adhering to the diet, you can lose up to one pound per day.

Most people can afford to lighten up their load and lose a few pounds. Those at their ideal body weight who lose a few pounds will regain the weight easily in the Detoxification and Maintenance Diet plans. And you will gain your weight back with nutrients that are far superior to what you have eliminated. So, for the great majority, losing a few pounds is not something to be concerned about.

For those who are so fragile that a 2- to 5-pound weight loss can make a major difference between the right energy level or feeling weak and sick, invariably 3 to 6 months need be spent on the Hi·Lite Maintenance Diet plan before beginning the cleansing process. Then, when the reserve of your body energy stores has been built up for a while, go back and enjoy the benefits of the Cleansing Diet.

THE RISKS OF THE CLEANSING DIET

For those individuals in good health, there are essentially no risks on the Hi·Lite Cleansing Diet. For the person in less than optimal health (nutritional "twilight zone"), the greatest risk is that you will get clear and find out within the week just how unwell you really are. Be assured, that a low-protein cleansing vegetarian diet is a sound starting point to gaining back your sanity. The kind of change the Hi·Lite Cleansing Diet makes in your lifestyle are all for the better. They are akin to spending time in a winter setting, in the mountains, the snow, the cold, the sunshine, the fresh air, seashore, or fresh streams, creeks, or rivers. The fact is that by slowing down your life and getting involved in the experience of the Cleansing Diet, you beneficially raise your consciousness and feed your well-being.

During the cleansing process, a variety of new and interesting experiences can take place. There are some individuals who from beginning to finish actually experience nothing but total euphoric well-being. Then there are many who experience euphoria 85-90% of the time and at other times find themselves a bit unfamiliar with their new slowed-down space and time consciousness. Some will have a few intermittent attacks of fatigue or fear of the unknown. And yet there are others that are plagued with foul body odors, catarrhal elimination, headaches, toxic skin eruptions, joint discomforts, and strange tastes in their mouths.

What happens really is very individualized and is determined by your metabolic efficiency. When you have earned the best of health, you'll experience minimal to none of the potential side effects of going on the Hi·Lite Cleansing Diet. Those of you whose health is most fragile will usually experience the most discomfort. And, it is important to work through these phases for short periods of time to move onto a higher level of physiological integrity, universal consciousness, and strength of emotional character. It sort of reminds me of the runner who reaches a mile and a half and feels weak and tired. He can experience some growth and development by just pushing ahead a little bit until he is in better shape, at which point he will be able to tolerate a two-mile run with great ease. Those, of course, in the best of health will experience nothing but joy and light on the Cleansing Diet.

Bear in mind that it is not uncommon in some 15-50% of patients to report some weakness and fatigue at one or two points in the first four days of cleansing. Invariably, as cellular poisons are broken up and broken loose, they pour into your circulation. This can commonly cause you to feel a lack of total well-being. Do not fret. It is temporary. To overcome the tired, often drugged-like feeling, you simply have to slow down the cleansing process by simply adding some *protein* to your program. For example, by adding 1½ Tbsp. of brewers yeast to fresh juice, or by devouring some extra celery stalks with unsalted peanut butter or almond butter, you raise the protein level sufficiently to slow down the cleansing and slow down your tired feelings. Most of the time, you can prevent getting tired by recharging your Hi·Lite mind with meditation and tuning up your body with physical exercise before each meal. Also, taking the proper vitamins and getting enough rest cuts back any potential side effects of the Cleansing Diet. Cut it up and cut it loose. Know that mentally it is up to you to recharge the will power of your Hi·Lite mind and rise to the occasion. With consistent positive thinking you can work through these tougher periods and make them very temporary.

For those who experience a splitting headache from the volcanic action of explosive negative energy that is released in the Cleansing Diet, there are two natural remedies. The first is hydrotherapy, that is, to immerse yourself in a natural fresh cold water source, such as the ocean, or take a cold shower and direct the cold water to your forehead. You will find the headache will disappear. The other solution is to go to bed. Sleep, help! When you awake your headache will be gone. And, by doing some acupressure on the main headache points of the body along the large intestine (LI-4) and the gall bladder (GB-20) meridians, you can often induce the headache to disappear. Sometimes 600 mg. of calcium lactate and 100 mg. of B-6, taken together, will do away with the headaches. Neck adjustment, massage, and acupuncture can also help.

The 21·Day Del Mar Diet

NUTRITIONAL SUPPLEMENTS
FOR THE CLEANSING DIET

In effect to minimize any potential side effects from the Cleansing Diet, be sure you are taking the proper vitamins and nutritional supplements.

VITAMIN E (mixed tocopherols)	400 I.U. one time with your fruit juice 15 minutes before breakfast
VITAMIN B-1	100 mg. one time a day (at breakfast)
VITAMIN B-6	100 mg. one time a day (at breakfast)
HI-POTENCY B-COMPLEX Super B, Mega B)	one with each meal
VITAMIN C	1000 mg. two times a day (at breakfast and at dinner time)
FOLIC ACID	2 mg. one time a day
VITAMIN B-12	1000 mcg. once a day
BREWERS YEAST	1½ Tbsp. twice a day blended in juice and taken between meals for a pick-up

With the exception of Vitamin E and brewers yeast, your vitamins are to be taken with the smallest amount of juice, tea, or water in the middle of your meal.

Rarely but sometimes, your tired feeling comes from being over-alkalined because your condition is already alkaline, and now you are going on a more alkaline Hi·Lite Cleansing program. In this situation, some acid-forming foods are in order. Usually a couple of tablets of hydrochloric acid along with acid-forming peanut butter will alleviate the feeling. You can tell whether your body is over-alkaline or not by checking the urine with phenaphtazine paper. When the urine PH is 7 or greater, your body is in an alkaline state, and I suggest you eat more acid-forming foods while on your Cleansing Diet. Take the first specimen in the morning.

Vomiting, dizziness, fatigue, lethargy, and lightheadedness may come and go on a cleansing diet. And anyone who sustains these symptoms after a week of cleansing needs for certain to be under the care of a qualified supervising physician. In fact, don't be afraid to ask your primary physician to check you out and supervise your cleansing. Who knows, maybe you will be able to get him to go on it with you.

In summary, the main risks of the Hi·Lite Cleansing Diet are for those who are malnourished or hypoglycemic. These individuals can experience a metabolic stress which will further weaken their system. When you are too weak to comfortably withstand *generating enough vital energy on your own,* it is not advised at this juncture to be on a cleansing diet. When you are that food dependent, you need first to build up your body. Once it is substantially reconstructed, you can then begin a cleansing program.

Another important risk to keep in consideration is for those who stay on a cleansing diet for too long. Individuals can overcleanse by staying on a cleansing diet for longer than three weeks. At this point, you can run into protein malnutrition, calcium deficiencies, and iron deficiencies. As noted, seven days usually is sufficient.

The great majority on the Hi·Lite Cleansing Diet have brisk increased bowel movement during the cleansing program. In fact, it is not uncommon to eliminate some three to six times a day. It is because all the fresh vegetables and fruits are beginning to purge your intestines. Cleansing means cleansing the intestines as well.

SEDENTARY COLON SYNDROME

Interestingly, there are some people who find that they can get constipated on a cleansing diet in spite of the increase of roughage in their diet. For these people, the tone in their intestinal tract is less than optimal. Inability to respond to a higher fiber diet indicates colonic lethargy. This is often the result of a sedentary burned out lifestyle of high emotional stress, refined junk foods, and insufficient exercise. It is the *sedentary colon syndrome.* In these individuals, the elimination of poisons and garbage is sometimes slower than their accumulation of it. In other words, those individuals whose colons are responding to higher fiber diets with a slower pattern of bowel movements need to turn to a Detoxification Diet and add more grains and fibers to their diet, first. When there are still no results after two weeks on the Detoxification Diet, it is advised to go onto the maintenance program. Results mean that the frequency of bowel movements approach at least one and sometimes up to two a day.

IT TAKES POSITIVE HI·LITE ENERGY
TO RELEASE DARK NEGATIVE ENERGY

In addition to serving as a catalyst to your overall wellness process, the Hi·Lite Cleansing Diet will instantly create changes in your life and lifestyle. After one week on the Cleansing Diet, your assimilation will be improved. In summary, the Cleansing Diet will:

- Purify your mind and body.

- Initiate the momentum to sustain a total bodily cleansing.

- Encourage merriment and nutrition for the heart and soul.

- Raise your consciousness,

- Metabolically change the body chemistry to a more alkaline state.

- Activate the wellness process of total healing.

- Reconnect your thoughts, feelings, and body to your soul.

- Turn in negative toxic energies for positive, new life-enhancing energy.

- Bring about effective weight loss.

- Rejuvenate positive, loving emotions.

It is a wonderful opportunity to learn the slow, relaxed mental discipline of good eating habits.

CONCLUSION

You have the option to choose a number of different fruit and vegetable combinations to meet your needs on the Cleansing Diet. For those who like to experience a wide variety of taste, color, textures, and sensations, feel free to create your own selection within the scope of the rules and guidelines. Keep in mind at all times that as long as you stay within the rules and guidelines of the Hi·Lite Cleansing Diet you will kick your field goal and score. In fact, you can choose any of the fresh fruit salads from the FRUIT SALAD SUPREMES, or raw vegetable salads from the LEAFY-GREEN CHLOROPHYLL SALADS, and repeat them with some frequency and still enjoy them. For example, many patients enjoy eating melon salads nearly every morning during the summer and citrus salads in the winter. Although variety is recommended, don't feel that you must vary each and every day. Variety is very individualized. Realize that there is a lot of variety within every one of your food groupings already. Most people find that by varying the salad dressings on the raw vegetable salads they can truly enjoy two basic leafy-green vegetable salads every day.

Your study of human nutrition begins with *you* as you put together for yourself your New Age cosmic diet. Today, the tap water is chemically polluted. So is the air. And it is basic to realize that mountain air is better than polluted air and that fresh water is better than polluted water. The time is right to acknowledge that fresh natural foods are superior to polluted foods. Keep in mind, it is the *quality in your diet*, not just what you eat that really counts. Are you ready to revolutionize your eating habits? It will not be difficult for you to find out how your diet can most positively influence your consciousness.

HI·LITE CLEANSING BREAKFAST (7:00·8:00 a.m.)

Spring:
(1) Papaya-pineapple juice (6 oz.)
15 minutes later:
(2) **SOUTH AMERICAN TROPICAL FRUIT SALAD**
• Papaya, ½ cup
• Pineapple, ½ cup
• Banana, 1 medium
Raw or roasted almonds (15-25)
Alfalfa sprouts (as many as you want)

Summer:
(1) Watermelon juice (6 oz.)
15 minutes later:
(2) **SUMMER MELON SALAD**
• Canteloupe, ½ medium
• Watermelon, ½ cup
• Honeydew, ½ cup
Raw or roasted almonds (15-25)
Alfalfa sprouts (as many as you want)

Autumn:
(1) Apple juice (6 oz.)
15 minutes later:
(2) **WALDORF APPLE SALAD AMBROSIA**
• Pippin apple, ½ medium
• Pear, ½ medium
• Banana, 1 medium
Raw or roasted almonds (15-25)
Alfalfa sprouts (as many as you want)

Winter:
(1) Orange juice (6 oz.)
15 minutes later:
(2) **WINTER CITRUS SALAD**
• Orange, 1 medium
• Pink grapefruit, ½ medium
• Pineapple, ½ cup
Raw or roasted almonds (15-25)
Alfalfa sprouts (as many as you want)

HI·LITE CLEANSING LUNCHEON (12:30·2:00 p.m.)

(1) Fresh carrot juice (6-8 oz.). *15 minutes later:*
(2) **GARDEN-GREEN CHLOROPHYLL SALAD**
• Romaine lettuce, 2-4 leaves   • Swiss chard, 1-2 leaves
• Spinach, 4 leaves   • Parsley, 1 Tbsp.
• Alfalfa sprouts, ½ cup   • Red onion, ¼ medium
• Tomato, ½ large   • Carrot, 1 medium
                • KELP-FROM-THE-SEA DRESSING
(3) 1-2 celery stalks with 1 Tbsp. crunchy, unsalted peanut butter
OR
(1) Fresh fruit juice in season (6 oz.). *15 minutes later:*
(2) **MELTZER FRUIT SALAD SUPREME** in season
(3) 2-3 oz. mixed nuts

HI·LITE CLEANSING DINNER (5:30·7:00 p.m.)

(1) Fresh carrot, carrot-celery, or carrot-celery-beet juice (8 oz.). *15 minutes later:*
(2) **SPICE-OF-LIFE SPINACH SALAD**
• Spinach, 4 leaves   • Alfalfa sprouts, ½ cup
• Romaine lettuce, 2-4 leaves   • Red onion, ¼ medium
• Tomato, ½ large   • Celery, 1 stalk
                • ITALIAN HERBAL DRESSING
                • Sunflower seeds, 2 tsp.
(3) BROCCOLI-ZUCCHINI VEGETABLE PLATTER
• Broccoli, ½ cup
• Zucchini, ½ cup
• String beans, ½ cup
(4) SPANISH BAKED POTATO (1 medium baked potato with CLEANSING CHILI SAUCE).

HI·LITE CLEANSING BREAKFAST (7:00 · 8:00 a.m.)

Spring:
(1) Orange juice (6 oz.)
  15 minutes later
(2) **ZESTY SPRING SALAD**
  • Pineapple, ½ cup
  • Banana, 1 medium
  • Strawberries, 5 large
  Raw or roasted almonds (15-25)
  Alfalfa sprouts (as many as you want)

Summer:
(1) Watermelon juice (6 oz.)
  15 minutes later:
(2) **SUMMER MELON SALAD**
  • Cantaloupe, ½ medium
  • Watermelon, ½ cup
  • Honeydew, ½ cup
  Raw or roasted almonds (15-25)
  Alfalfa sprouts (as many as you want)

Autumn:
(1) Pear juice (6 oz.)
  15 minutes later:
(2) *MIXED APPLE SALAD*
  • Pippin apple, ½ medium
  • Macintosh apple, ½ medium
  • Golden Delicious apple, ½ medium
  Raw or roasted almonds (15-25)
  Alfalfa sprouts (as many as you want)

Winter:
(1) Orange juice (6 oz.)
  15 minutes later:
(2) **ORANGE WONDERLAND SALAD**
  • Orange, ½ medium
  • Pineapple, ½ cup
  • Banana, ½ medium
  Raw or roasted almonds (15-25)
  Alfalfa sprouts (as many as you want)

HI·LITE CLEANSING LUNCHEON (12:30 · 2:00 p.m.)

(1) Fresh carrot juice (6-8 oz.), *15 minutes later:*
(2) **SPROUTED GARDEN·FRESH DINNER SALAD**
  • Romaine lettuce, 2-4 leaves
  • Tomato, ½ large
  • Alfalfa sprouts, ½ cup
  • Red cabbage, ¼ cup
  • Parsley, 1 Tbsp.
  • Red onion, ¼ medium
  • Carrot, 1 medium
    • LEMON-GARLIC DRESSING
(3) 1-2 celery stalks with 1 Tbsp. crunchy, unsalted peanut butter

OR

(1) Fresh fruit juice in season (6 oz.), *15 minutes later:*
(2) **MELTZER FRIUT SALAD SUPREME** in season
(3) 2-3 oz. mixed nuts

HI·LITE CLEANSING DINNER (5:30 · 7:00 p.m.)

(1) Fresh carrot, carrot-celery, or carrot-celery-beet juice (8 oz.)
  15 minutes later:
(2) **RAW MUSHROOM SALAD**
  • Romaine lettuce, 4 leaves
  • Sprouts, ½ cup
  • Tomato, ½ large
  • Mushrooms, 10 small or 4 large
  • Cucumber, six 1/8 inch slices
  • Celery, 1 stalk
    • LEMON-VINAIGRETTE DRESSING
    • Sesame or sunflower seeds, 2 tsp.
(3) STEAMED ASPARAGUS-BROCCOLI MEDLEY
  • Asparagus, 5-6 spears
  • Broccoli, ½ cup
  • Zucchini, ½ cup
(4) CORN ON THE COB with CLEANSING CHILI SAUCE.

HI·LITE NUTRITIONAL CLEANSING: DAY 3
BREAK · IT · DOWN: CLEAN IT OUT

HI·LITE CLEANSING BREAKFAST (7:00-8:00 a.m.)

Spring:
(1) Papaya juice (6 oz.)
   15 minutes later:
(2) **MANGO DAYBREAK DELIGHT**
   • Mango, ½ medium
   • Banana, ½ medium
   • Pineapple, ½ cup
   Raw or roasted almonds (15-25)
   Alfalfa sprouts (as many as you want)

Autumn:
(1) Apple juice (6 oz.)
   15 minutes later:
(2) **AUTUMN ENERGY SALAD**
   • Pippin apple, ½ medium
   • Papaya, ½ cup
   • Banana, 1 medium
   Raw or roasted almonds (15-25)
   Alfalfa sprouts (as many as you want)

Summer:
(1) Papaya juice (6 oz.)
   15 minutes later:
(2) **CHERRY·FRIAR PLUM SALAD**
   • Cherries, 8
   • Friar plum, 1
   • Nectarine, 1 medium (or other variety of plum)
   Raw or roasted almonds (15-25)
   Alfalfa sprouts (as many as you want)

Winter:
(1) **Grapefruit juice (6 oz.)**
   15 minutes later:
(2) **PAPAYA PARADISE SALAD**
   • Orange, ½ medium
   • Papaya, ½ cup
   • Banana, 1 medium
   Raw or roasted almonds (15-25)
   Alfalfa sprouts (as many as you want)

HI·LITE CLEANSING LUNCHEON (12:30-2:00 p.m.)

(1) Fresh carrot juice (6-8 oz.), *15 minutes later:*
(2) **COOL CUCUMBER SALAD**
   • Romaine lettuce, 4 leaves
   • Alfalfa sprouts, ½ cup
   • Tomato, ½ large
   • Radishes, 2 small
   • Celery, 1 stalk
   • Cucumber, six ½ inch slices
   • Green pepper, ¼ large
      • AVOCADO GREEN DRESSING
(1) 1-2 celery stalks with 1 Tbsp. crunchy, unsalted peanut butter.

OR

(1) Fresh fruit juice in season (6 oz.), *15 minutes later:*
(2) **MELTZER FRUIT SALAD SUPREME** in season
(3) 2-3 oz. mixed nuts

HI·LITE CLEANSING DINNER (5:30-7:00 p.m.)

(1) Fresh carrot, carrot-celery, or carrot-celery-beet juice (8 oz.)
   15 minutes later:
(2) **SUPER SPROUT SALAD**
   • Bean sprouts, all you want
   • Alfalfa sprouts, all you want
   • Sunflower seed sprouts, all you want
   • Romaine lettuce, 4 leaves
   • Tomato, ½ large
   • Red onion, ¼ cup
      • HERBAL VINAIGRETTE DRESSING
      • Sesame or sunflower seeds, 2 tsp.
(3) BROCCOLI-MIXED GREENS VEGETABLE SOUP
(4) BAKED POTATO with CLEANSING CHILI SAUCE

BREAK · IT · LOOSE: EXCHANGE THE LIGHT FOR
FOR THE DARK

HI·LITE CLEANSING BREAKFAST (7:00 · 8:00 a.m.)

Spring:
(1) Papaya-pineapple juice (6 oz.)
    15 minutes later:
(2) **CHERRY SUPREME SALAD**
    • Cherries, 8
    • Peach, 1 medium
    • Banana, 1 medium
    Raw or roasted almonds (15-25)
    Alfalfa sprouts (as many as you want)

Autumn:
(1) Apple juice (6 oz.)
    15 minutes later:
(2) **PEACEFUL PEAR SALAD**
    • Pear, 1 medium
    • Papaya, 1 cup
    • Banana, 1 medium
    Raw or roasted almonds (15-25)
    Alfalfa sprouts (as many as you want)

Summer:
(1) Papaya juice (6 oz.)
    15 minutes later:
(2) **APRICOT SUNSHINE SALAD**
    • Apricots, 3 medium
    • Peach, 1 medium
    • Plum, 1 medium (or 8 cherries or 1 cup seedless green grapes)
    Raw or roasted almonds (15-25)
    Alfalfa sprouts (as many as you want)

Winter:
(1) Orange juice (6 oz.)
    15 minutes later:
(2) PINK GRAPEFRUIT WINTER SALAD
    • Pink grapefruit, ½ medium
    • Orange, ½ medium
    • Banana, 1 medium
    Raw or roasted almonds (15-25)
    Alfalfa sprouts (as many as you want)

HI·LITE CLEANSING LUNCHEON (12:30 · 2:00 p.m.)

(1) Fresh carrot juice (6-8 oz.), *15 minutes later:*
(2) **MEXICAN CABBAGE SALAD**
    • Red cabbage, ¼ cup   • Romaine lettuce, 4 leaves
    • Green cabbage, ¼ cup   • Alfalfa sprouts, ½ cup
    • Red onion, ¼ cup   • Tomato, ½ large
              • LEMON-GARLIC DRESSING
(3) 1-2 celery stalks with 1 Tbsp. crunchy, unsalted peanut butter

OR

(1) Fresh fruit juice in season
(2) **MELTZER FRUIT SALAD SUPREME** in season
(3) 2-3 oz. mixed nuts

HI·LITE CLEANSING DINNER (5:30 · 7:00 p.m.)

(1) Fresh carrot, carrot-celery or carrot-celery-beet juice (8 oz.)
    15 minutes later:
(2) **CUCUMBER-BEET SALAD**
    • Romaine lettuce, 4 leaves   • Tomato, ½ large
    • Cucumber   • Alfalfa sprouts, ½ cup
    • Raw shredded beet, ½ medium • Carrot, 1 small
              • ITALIAN DRESSING
           • Sesame or sunflower seeds, 2 tsp.
(3) CHINESE STEAMED VEGETABLE COMBINATION
    • Chinese snow peas, 1 cup   • Jicama, ¼ cup
    • Bok choy, 1 cup   • Carrot, 1 small

HI·LITE CLEANSING BREAKFAST (7:00 · 8:00 a.m.)

Spring:
(1) Papaya juice (6 oz.)
   15 minutes later:
(2) **GRAPE DELIGHT SALAD**
   • Seedless green grapes, 1 cup
   • Red grapes, ½ cup
   • Concord grapes, ½ cup
   Raw or roasted almonds (15-25)
   Alfalfa sprouts (as many as you want)

Autumn:
(1) Pear juice (6 oz.)
   15 minutes later:
(2) **WALDORF APPLE SALAD AMBROSIA**
   • Pippin apple, 1 medium
   • Pear, ½ medium
   • Banana, 1 medium
   Raw or roasted almonds (15-25)
   Alfalfa sprouts (as many as you want)

Summer:
(1) Papaya juice (6 oz.)
   15 minutes later:
(2) **HAWAIIAN FRUIT SALAD**
   • Papaya, ½ cup
   • Mango, ½ medium
   • Pinapple, ½ cup
   Raw or roasted almonds (15-25)
   Alfalfa sprouts (as many as you want)

Winter:
(1) Orange juice (6 oz.)
   15 minutes later:
(2) **SOUTH AMERICAN TROPICAL FRUIT SALAD**
   • Pineapple, ½ cup
   • Papaya, ½ cup
   • Banana, 1 medium
   Raw or roasted almonds (15-25)
   Alfalfa sprouts (as many as you want)

HI·LITE CLEANSING LUNCHEON (12:30 · 2:00 p.m.)

(1) Fresh carrot juice (6-8 oz.), *15 minutes later:*
(2) AVOCADO-TOMATO GRANDE SALAD
   • Avocado, ½ medium
   • Tomato, ½ large
   • Celery, 1 stalk
   • Romaine lettuce, 4 leaves
   • Alfalfa sprouts, ½ cup
   • Carrot, 1 medium
      • RED CAYENNE DRESSING
(3) 1-2 celery stalks with 1 Tbsp. crunchy, unsalted peanut butter

OR

(1) Fresh fruit juice in season (6 oz.), *15 minutes later:*
(2) **MELTZER FRUIT SALAD SUPREME** in season
(3) 2-3 oz. mixed nuts

HI·LITE CLEANSING DINNER (5:30 · 7:00 p.m.)

(1) Fresh carrot, carrot-celery, or carrot-celery-beet juice (8 oz.)
   15 minutes later:
(2) **SPICE-OF-LIFE SPINACH SALAD**
   • Spinach, 4 leaves
   • Romaine lettuce, 2-4 leaves
   • Tomato, ½ large
   • Alfalfa sprouts, ½ cup
   • Red onion, ¼ medium
   • Celery, 1 stalk
      • ONION-GARLIC DRESSING
      • Sesame or sunflower seeds, 2 tsp.
(3) CAULIFLOWER MIXED VEGETABLE PLATTER
   • Zucchini, 1 cup
   • Cauliflower, ½ cup
   • Broccoli, ½ cup
(4) BAKED YAM, 1 medium, garnished with fresh parsley

HI·LITE CLEANSING BREAKFAST (7:00 - 8:00 a.m.)

Spring:
(1) Orange juice (6 oz.)
15 minutes later:
(2) **SOUTH AMERICAN TROPICAL FRUIT SALAD**
• Papaya, ½ cup
• Banana, 1 medium
• Pineapple, ½ cup
Raw or roasted almonds (15-25)
Alfalfa sprouts (as many as you want)

Autumn:
(1) apple juice (6 oz.)
15 minutes later:
(2) **AUTUMN ENERGY SALAD**
• Pippin apple, ½ medium
• Papaya, ½ cup
• Banana, 1 medium
Raw or roasted almonds (15-25)
Alfalfa sprouts (as many as you want)

Summer:
(1) Papaya juice (6 oz.)
15 minutes later:
(2) **NECTARINE-PEACH SALAD**
• Nectarine, 1 medium
• Peach, 1 medium
• Cherries, 8
Raw or roasted almonds (15-25)
Alfalfa sprouts (as many as you want)

Winter:
(1) Orange juice (6 oz.)
15 minutes later:
(2) **PINK GRAPEFRUIT WINTER SALAD**
• Pink grapefruit, ½ medium
• Orange, ½ medium
• Banana, 1 medium
Raw or roasted almonds (15-25)
Alfalfa sprouts (as many as you want)

HI·LITE CLEANSING LUNCHEON (12:30 - 2:00 p.m.)

(1) Fresh carrot juice (6-8 oz.), *15 minutes later:*
(2) **RADIANT RADISH SALAD**
• Romaine lettuce, 4 leaves
• Alfalfa sprouts, ½ cup
• Tomato, ½ large
• Radishes, 2 small
• Red onion, ¼ cup
• Chopped parsley, 1 Tbsp.
• HERBAL ITALIAN DRESSING
(3) 1-2 celery stalks with 1 Tbsp. crunchy, unsalted peanut butter

OR

(1) Fresh fruit juice in season (6 oz.), *15 minutes later:*
(2) **MELTZER FRUIT SALAD SUPREME** in season
(3) 2-3 oz. mixed nuts

HI·LITE CLEANSING DINNER (5:30 - 7:00 p.m.)

(1) Fresh carrot, carrot-celery, or carrot-celery-beet juice (8 oz.)
15 minutes later:
(2) **JICAMA-BEET TREAT**
• Jicama, ½ cup
• Raw grated beet, ½ medium
• Carrot, 1 small
• Romaine lettuce, 4 leaves
• Tomato, ½ large
• Alfalfa sprouts, ½ cup
• KELP-FROM-THE-SEA DRESSING
• Sesame or sunflower seeds, 2 tsp.
(3) BRUSSEL SPROUT-MIXED VEGETABLE PLATTER
• Brussel sprouts, 1 cup
• Zucchini, ½ cup
• Green pepper, ¼ cup
(4) BAKED POTATO with CLEANSING CHILI SAUCE

HI·LITE CLEANSING BREAKFAST (7:00 - 8:00 a.m.)

Spring:
(1) Pineapple juice (6 oz.)
15 minutes later:
(2) **ZESTY SPRING SALAD**
 • Pineapple, ½ cup
 • Banana, 1 medium
 • Strawberries, 5 large
 Raw or roasted almonds (15-25)
 Alfalfa sprouts (as many as you want)

Autumn:
(1) Apple juice (6 oz.)
15 minutes later:
(2) **GRAPE CURE SALAD**
 • Mono grape diet of seedless Thompson green grapes, or red grapes, 1 to 2 cups at a time
 Raw or roasted almonds (15-25)
 Alfalfa sprouts (as many as you want)

Summer:
(1) Papaya juice (6 oz.)
15minutes later:
(2) **MANGO PEACH SALAD**
 • Mango, ½ medium
 • Peach, 1 medium
 • Banana, ½ medium
 Raw or roasted almonds (15-25)
 Alfalfa sprouts (as many as you want)

Winter:
(1) Pineapple juice (6 oz.)
15 minutes later:
(2) **PAPAYA PARIDISE SALAD**
 • Orange, ½ medium
 • Papaya, ½ cup
 • Banana, 1 medium
 Raw or roasted almonds (15-25)
 Alfalfa sprouts (as many as you want)

HI·LITE CLEANSING LUNCHEON (12:30 - 2:00 p.m.)

(1) Fresh carrot juice (6-8 oz.), *15 minutes later:*
(2) **BASIC AVOCADO SALAD**
 • Avocado, ½ medium
 • Raw Shredded beet, ½ medium
 • Romaine lettuce, 4 leaves
 • Tomato, ½ large
 • Alfalfa sprouts, ½ cup
 • **HERBAL ITALIAN DRESSING**
(3) 1-2 celery stalks with 1 Tbsp. crunchy, unsalted peanut butter

OR

(1) Fresh fruit juice in season (6 oz.), *15 minutes later:*
(2) **MELTZER FRUIT SALAD SUPREME** in season
(3) 2-3 oz. mixed nuts

HI·LITE CLEANSING DINNER (5:30 - 7:00 p.m.)

(1) Fresh carrot, carrot-celery, or carrot-celery-beet juice (8 oz.)
15 minutes later:
(2) **GARDEN PEA SALAD**
 • Chinese snow peas, 12
 • Romaine lettuce, 4 leaves
 • Green peas, 2 Tbsp.
 • Green pepper, ½ large
 • Alfalfa sprouts, ½ cup
 • Tomato, ½ large
 • **ONION-GARLIC DRESSING**
 • Sesame or sunflower seeds, 2 tsp.
(3) BROCCOLI-MIXED GREENS VEGETABLE SOUP
(4) CORN ON THE COB with CLEANSING CHILI SAUCE

3: THE CLEANSING DIET RECIPES

ORGANIZING YOUR HEALTH FOOD KITCHEN

Your diet is the foundation of your journey towards enhanced health. As with any new experience, a certain amount of practical knowledge and organization is called for. Correct timing also goes into developing a rhythmic approach towards healthful, wholesome food preparation.

Preparing your food in a clean, well-organized kitchen can make it more pleasurable and enjoyable. Remember, your kitchen is a healing center for building up your health. Appropriate Light and green plants help create the right environment. You will need to have the correct tools and equipment in your health food kitchen.

THE ESSENTIALS

A *blender* can be used for making smoothies, delicious salad dressings, melon juice (blend melon and strain out the pulp), blending tomatoes for soups and sauces, and even for grinding nuts.

You need a *pot* with a *tight fitting lid* for cooking rice or other grains and another *larger covered pan* for soups and for steaming vegetables.

A *stainless steel vegetable steamer* is essential and can be purchased in most health food stores or supermarkets.

You need a *cutting board*. Some good *sharp knives* and assorted silverware are necessary. A *grater*, *measuring cup*, *strainer*, *garlic press*, *sprouting jar*, *casserole dish*, and *jars or containers* with tight fitting lids for storing nuts, seeds and grains are recommended.

Wooden spoons and chop sticks add a practical and aesthetic value to cooking and dining. Eating with chop sticks will enable you to eat more slowly.

Fresh vegetable and fruit juices can usually be purchased at health food stores. Eventually you may want to purchase a *juicer* to assure freshness and high quality. The Champion juicer seems to be the best juicer for its versatility. You can make fresh fruit and vegetable juices, finely shred vegetables for nut loafs and vegetable burgers and also make nut butters with it.

A *wok* is excellent for sauteing vegetables to maintain the highest nutritional value. A covered frying pan can be used in place of a wok.

A *colander* is essential for draining pasta and comes in handy when washing vegetables.

Cast iron cookware is sturdy and lasts a lifetime. It is superb for sauteing vegetables because it requires little or no oil. Avoid aluminum cookware because of its toxic health hazards. The same is true of pans with non-stick coatings. With wear, the coating breaks down and may chip off into the food. Play it safe and stick with cast iron, stainless steel, clay and glass pyrex-type cookware.

Other essential equipment would include the following:

Measuring spoons	Mortar and pestle
Liquid measuring cup	Manual spice grinder
Dry measuring cup	Teapot
Spatula	Vegetable peeler
Tongs	Vegetable brush
Soup ladle	Pastry brush
Masher	Toaster
Wire shick	

THE EXTRAS

Many innovative cooking appliances have come on the market in the past few years. The *food processor* is one of the most popular. It can be very useful when chopping vegetables for a large family, along with its other varied uses such as blending, kneading bread dough, grating cheese, chopping nuts, mixing dressings, and pureeing vegetables.

A *crock pot* can be an extra bonus for the working cook. Soups, stews, and beans can be started in the morning and be ready for a relaxed evening meal.

Nut grinders are useful when you find yourself grinding large quantities of nuts. Nevertheless, a good quality blender can do the same process.

A *toaster oven* can be a valuable tool when melting cheese on tortillas or toasted bread, making "pita pizzas" (see page 138), or for simply making toast. It's most important contribution is its conservation of energy.

Pressure cookers are time and energy savers when preparing beans and soybeans. Be sure your pressure cooker is in good work-

ing condition. Check the valve on the top to make certain it's working properly. Follow instructions for cooking time and pressure
according to your individual type of cooker.

Microwave ovens are not recommended because of their extreme
high heat.

Look in any kitchenware store and you will be amazed at the
variety of different equipment. The main guide is to begin cooking
with whatever basics you have. Then add the extras, depending upon
which items will get the most use.

HERBS AND SPICES

The best way to learn how to use herbs is by personal experience
and experimentation. Use the following as a guideline:

Basil — Goes well with tomatoes and tomato sauce. For Italian
food use onions and garlic and equal amounts of basil and
oregano and a smaller amount of thyme.

Bay leaves — Use one or two leaves whenever you're making
soup or cooking rice or beans. Remove leaves before serving.
Tastes good in Italian sauces.

Cayenne — Use this herb sparingly and then taste or place on
the table so each person can season individually. Cayenne is
used in Mexican and Indian dishes and is very hot and spicy.

Celery seed — Can be used in salads, soups, salad dressings, nut
loafs.

Chili powder — Use with restraint. Add a little at a time. Then
taste before adding more. Use in beans, soups, Mexican dishes.

Chives — Make a flavorful garnish to salads, soups, or main
dishes.

Cinnamon — For sprinkling on fruit salads, hot apple cider or
making desserts.

Cloves — Used in curries and soups. Also in hot apple cider.

Coriander — A spice used in chili powder and curry. Use in
curries, beans and soups.

Cumin — Adds spice to Indian and Mexican dishes.

Curry — Is not an herb but is actually a blend of spices and
seasonings. Use curry in Indian dishes, i.e., curried lentils,
vegetable curry.

Dill — Sprinkle on salads, use in salad dressings and soups or
with potatoes.

Fennel seeds — For use in breads, Italian dishes.

Garlic — Keep fresh garlic on hand to use in soups, salad dressings, and main dishes. A garlic press makes this pungent herb much easier to use.

Ginger — For Oriental cooking and adding to sauteed vegetables.

Marjoram — For soups, stews, salads, spaghetti sauces, vegetables, nutloafs.

Mint — For sauces, beverages, and as herb teas.

Nutmeg — Used similarly and in conjunction with cinnamon and cloves.

Onion — Another food to keep on hand for addition to sauteed vegetables, soups, and other main dishes. Green onions or scallions are best used in salads and as a garnish for soups. The yellow, white, or red onions are best for cooking.

Oregano — Use with basil, with tomatoes, and any Italian dishes.

Paprika — Use in salad dressings and sprinkled on potatoes and vegetables as a colorful garnish.

Parsley — Add to salad dressings, casseroles, soups, potatoes, carrots, squash, spreads, and sauces.

Rosemary — For soups and salad dressings.

Saffron — Use in brown rice to add variety of taste.

Sage — Add to nut loafs and soups.

Tarragon — For tomato sauces, french dressing, and salads.

Thyme — With basil and oregano in Italian dishes; add to soups, entrees.

Vanilla beans — To flavor nut milks and smoothies chop up ½ bean in blender.

STOCKING YOUR HI·LITE KITCHEN

Your next step is to stock up on the essential ingredients of the Meltzer Hi·Lite Diet. You may feel a bit overwhelmed when you visit the produce department in your local health food store or supermarket. The variety of fruits and vegetables can make for a jungle of confusion.

Rule No. 1 is *go prepared*. Arm yourself with a well-thought-out shopping list. Plan your menus for the week. Decide which foods you need. Then make a list of items you will need to purchase at the store. The following categories are a checklist to stimulate your memory for the foods you would need:

1. **Elixirs, tonics, and beverages:** Be sure to check your supply of bottled water, herbal teas, and juices before you take a trip to the store.

2. **Appetizers:** How is your supply of avocados, lemons, salsa, and celery? How about your supply of nut butters?

3. **Salads:** Check your Hi·Lite fruit combination lists for the fruit salads of your choice. Then check your refrigerator's supply of those fruits. Do you have enough fresh greens, firm tomatoes, crisp sprouts, light-colored mushrooms, and other raw vegetables?

4. **Salad dressings:** Be sure you have cold pressed safflower, sesame, and olive oils and all other herbs you need to keep your daily garden green salads appetizing.

5. **Soups and stews:** Do you have the vegetables, dried lentils, beans, peas, pasta, flavorings (herbs and bouillion), and thickeners necessary for savory soups?

6. **Grains, nuts and seeds:** Check your recipes. Do you have the basic vegetables, rice, and flour necessary? Are you equipped with enough cereal, granola, nuts and seeds?

7. **Desserts:** See recipes. Do you have honey and other needed spices?

STAPLES TO HAVE ON HAND

Dry Goods

2 lbs. whole wheat flour
2 lbs. soy flour
2 lbs. whole wheat pastry flour
1 lb. wheat bran
1 lb. brewer's yeast
2 lbs. brown rice

Legumes

1 lb. garbanzo beans (chick peas)
1 lb. pinto beans
1 lb. lentils
1 lb. mung beans (can be used for sprouting)
1 lb. split peas
1 lb. kidney beans
1 lb. soybeans

Vegetables and sprouts

Vegetables for salads
Vegetables for steaming
Potatoes
Sprouts for salads

Fruits

A variety of fruits for your fresh fruit salads

Oils and spreads

Safflower oil
Sesame oil
Olive oil
Sesame tahini
Peanut butter (unsalted)

The 21-Day Del Mar Diet

57

Seasonings		Nuts and seeds
Basil	Ginger	Sunflower seeds
Bay leaves	Marjoram	Sesame seeds
Cayenne	Mint	Almonds
Celery seed	Nutmeg	Cashews
Chili powder	Onion	
Chives	Oregano	**Beverages**
Cinnamon	Paprika	Herbal teas
Cloves	Parsley	Juices
Coriander	Rosemary	Water
Cumin	Saffron	
Curry	Sage	**Miscellaneous**
Dill	Tarragon	Chili sauce
Fennel seeds	Thyme	Guacamole ingredients
Garlic	Vanilla beans	Tofu
		Herbs and spices
		Nutritional supplements
		Bee pollen

RECIPES FROM THE HI·LITE KITCHEN

Cleansing Diet Recipes

The following pages include food preparation tips to assist you in following the Hi·Lite Cleansing Diet. Recipes are categorized by food groups according to the standards of the cleansing diet.

FOOD GROUPS IA and IIA: Juices and Herbal Teas

Fluid intake is vital to the Cleansing Diet. High quality, pure, natural fluids facilitate the body's natural cleansing processes. Juices are best when fresh and made from unadulterated wholesome fruits and vegetables. Bottled natural mineral springs water is clearly preferred over tap water. Mineral water is preferred over distilled water due to its high natural content of essential trace minerals for the body. A twist of lemon or lime can be added for a colorful, flavorful and cleansing touch to your favorite bottled water. Herbal teas are soothing and are a supportive part of the Cleansing Diet.

To make *herbal teas:*

1 Tbsp. dry herb tea leaves per cup

or

2 Tbsp. fresh herb tea leaves per cup

1. Bring water to a boil. Remove from heat.

2. Now add tea leaves.

3. Cover. Let steep for 10-20 minutes. Do not boil leaves.

4. Strain; serve hot or cold. Honey may be added for sweetener. Sun tea can be made in cold water by letting herbs heat up in the sun for 3-4 hours.

Popular herbal teas:

Peppermint — has a soothing effect on the digestive organs, especially the stomach and intestines.

Chamomile — has a relaxing effect on your nerves.

Rosehips — high in vitamin C to increase your resistance.

Avoid non-herbal teas. They are high in caffeine content. Caffeine has a stimulating drug-like effect on your brain, kidneys, heart, nerves, and adrenal glands. Suggested coffee substitutes: Chicory and roasted barley. Two brand names are Postum and Roastaroma. They are coffee substitutes made from grain.

FOOD GROUP I: Fruit Salads

Rinse off the fruit. Rinsing removes dirt, pesticide residues and preservative sprays from the fruit. Scrub with a vegetable brush to remove wax. Slice or chop fruits and colorfully arrange in a bowl.

Limit your fruit salads to three fresh fruits. As a rule of thumb, one bowl of fruit usually measures to be 1½ cups and approximately 150 calories. Follow the Compatible Fruit Combinations as detailed in your specific Hi·Lite fruit salad selections. Even though you may eat a similar fruit salad every morning, you can create variety by choosing different fruits and by changing the way you prepare the salad. Be sure to pay attention to eye appeal and color when preparing your fruit. A salad of golden apples and yellow pears can appear monotonous. Explore a variety of new fruit tastes. Are you aware of how many different kinds of pears there are? There are bosch, D-anjou, bartlett, and more. For example, add zest to your salads with colorful green pippin apples, bright oranges, or luscious purple concord grapes. Become a food connosieur and see what you like best. Mix chopped fruits and place on a bed of alfalfa sprouts or top your favorite fruit combo with sprouts. Get involved in your food selection and preparation.

FOOD GROUP II: Vegetable Salads

The three main ingredients to the Hi·Lite garden fresh vegetable salads are romaine lettuce, sprouts, and tomato.

Lettuce:	Separate the leaves from the stem by gently pulling them off. Wash each leaf carefully. Dry with paper towels. Store in an airtight container such as a plastic bag with a twist tie or a bowl with tight-fitting lid. Place a paper napkin or paper towel in the bottom of the bowl to absorb moisture and store in the crispest container of your refrigerator. This not only keeps the lettuce longer, but this initial preparation saves you time when preparing your salad later. Tear lettuce leaves and place in bowl.
Tomato:	Use firm, red, ripe tomatoes, either the sweet cherry or large beefsteak variety.
Other Raw Vegetables:	Choose 2-4 additional fresh raw vegetables. Pay attention to your color combinations. Consult the Cleansing Diet Hi·Lite Leafy Green Chlorophyll Salads for the specifics. You can vary your salad by the way you cut and slice or grate the other vegetables you add. The main variation comes in the use of different salad dressing.
Sprouts:	Rinse and drain sprouts before adding them to your salad. You can mix the sprouts with the lettuce and tomato or use them as a garnish.

Alfalfa seeds are easily sprouted by soaking 2 Tbsp. seeds in ½ cup water overnight. Place in a jar with a mesh or net lid (can be made or purchased at health food store). Save the soak water for soups, drink it, or give it to your pets or plants — it's highly nutritious. Rinse the sprouts at least two times a day and place upside down in your dish drainer or tilt to drain. The sprouts will be ready in 3-5 days. Drain well before storing. If they are not green enough, simply set them on a window sill away from direct light, and rotate jar. They can be stored in the refrigerator in air-tight container.

You can also sprout *lentils*, *garbanzos* (chick peas), *azuki beans*, and *mung beans* right in the same container with the alfalfa seeds. The mung sprouts will be ready when they are about ½″ long.

FOOD GROUP III: Steamed Vegetable Combinations

How to Steam Your Vegetables

It takes practice to be able to steam the vegetables so they are tender, but not overcooked. In general, steam the harder vegetables such as broccoli and cauliflower first and add the softer vegetables such as mushrooms and squash towards the end. Fill the pan with enough water, usually ½-¾'', to flush level with the bottom surface of the steamer. Place the steamer inside, and then cover until the water boils. Then add the vegetables, cover, and turn the heat to medium. Remove from heat before tender. Keep covered until you reach desired texture.

Emphasize broccoli, zucchini, and stringbeans in your Cleansing Diet.

Cleansing Mixed-Greens Soup

1 small bunch spinach
1 small bunch turnip greens
1 small bunch greens (mustard, collard, etc.) of your choice
½ lb. fresh broccoli
1 small zucchini, diced
1 stalk celery, chopped
1 large tomato, chopped
1 medium turnip, diced
1 small rutabaga, diced
3 cloves garlic

1 onion, diced
1 carrot, scraped and diced
¼ head red cabbage, shredded
1 medium beet, diced
2 quarts water
¼ tsp. oregano
¼ tsp. marjoram
¼ tsp. basil
¼ tsp. fresh cracked pepper
A **dash** of cayenne
1 bay leaf

Place the turnip, rutabaga, carrot, and beet in a deep soup pot with a small amount of water to cover. Simmer, covered, until the vegetables are partially tender. Then add all the remaining ingredients and simmer, covered, for approximately 40 minutes. Serves 8-10.

FOOD GROUP IV: Natural Starchy Carbohydrates

Baked Potatoes

For potatoes or yams, wash well and do not peel. Stick the center of the potato several times with a fork. Then place on the middle rack of a 350° oven. It usually takes 45 minutes to one hour. Stick with a fork to test for doneness.

For hard winter squash, wash and slice lengthwise. Then remove seeds and inside membrane. Place cut side down on a cookie sheet or in a casserole dish. Add ¼" water. Bake at 350° until tender. Test with a fork for doneness. You can also bake with cut side up basting lightly with oil and sprinkling with your favorite herbs or cinnamon.

FOOD GROUP V: Cleansing Diet Protein

Nuts, seeds, nut butter, sprouts, and avocados, along with your baked potatoes and corn, give you the essential amino acids you need on the Cleansing Diet.

FOOD GROUP VI: Mixed Nuts

Purchase only unsalted nut butters. Raw or roasted nuts are acceptable. Here is how you oven toast your nuts:

Place raw nuts in a pie plate or on a cookie sheet and toast lightly 10 minutes at 350°, stir frequently. Nuts will be crisp when cooled. Lower heat to 200° for 5 more minutes. Stir frequently.

FOOD GROUP VII: Salad Dressings

Listed below are several salad dressings to brighten up your taste buds and add variety to your fresh green garden cleansing salads:

Lemon Garlic Dressing

Juice of a lemon
Cloves
1 clove garlic, pressed

1 yellow onion, minced
1 tsp. oregano
½ tsp. kelp
1 tsp. basil

Shake well in covered container. Allow flavors to blend in refrigerator.

Vinegarette Dressing

2-3 Tbsp. apple cider vinegar
1 clove garlic, pressed
Juice of one lemon.

½ tsp. kelp
1 tsp. oregano
½ tsp. paprika
1 tsp. basil

Mix in blender. Refrigerate to blend flavors.

Italian Herbal Dressing

3 large tomatoes
½ peeled cucumber
1 yellow onion, chopped
1 clove garlic, chopped
1 tsp. celery seed

1 tsp. paprika
1 tsp. dill
2-3 Tbsp. apple cider vinegar
½ tsp. chervil

Mix above ingredients in a blender. Chill to allow flavors to blend.

Avocado Green Dressing

1 medium avocado, ripened
Juice of ½ lemon
1 clove garlic, pressed

½ tsp. tamari or Spike seasoning
   to taste
1 pinch cayenne (optional)

Mix in blender.

Cleansing Chili Sauce

3 tomatoes
1 green pepper
½ tsp. oregano

1/8 tsp. red cayenne pepper
¼ cup green onions
1-2 tsp. chili powder

Put all ingredients in blender or food processor. Blend until tomatoes and
pepper are chopped coarsely.

Kelp-from-the-Sea Dressing

2-3 Tbsp. apple cider vinegar
1 clove garlic, pressed
1 yellow onion, minced

½ tsp. kelp
1 tsp. oregano
½ tsp. tamari sauce

Shake well in covered container. Allow flavors to blend in refrigerator.

Dynamic Herbal Dressing

⅔ cup lemon juice
3 scallions, chopped
¼ cup parsley, minced
½ tsp. celery seed

½ tsp. paprika
½ tsp. basil
1/8 tsp. each oregano, rosemary

Mix and chill one hour before serving.

Pyne's Cleansing Parsley Picante

1 cup parsley, chopped
6 green onions, sliced
1 tomato, diced
1 cup water
½ cup apple cider vinegar

1 tsp. kelp
2 cloves garlic, crushed
1 tsp. dill
1 green chile, baked and diced
 (include seeds)

Mix together and store in refrigerator.

Wholly Guacamole

At lunch time this Wholly Guacamole recipe is one option to accompany a fresh green garden salad.

1-2 medium avocadoes, ripe
Juice from ½ lemon
Chopped red onion, as desired
1 pinch red cayenne pepper (optional) —
 · Be careful — it's HOT

2-3 Tbsp. salsa (optional)
Chopped, fresh, green chilies —
 seeds removed (the seeds are
 the hottest part)*

Smash avocado with fork. Mix in other ingredients. Serve on top of a vegetable salad in place of salad dressing, or use as a dip for celery stalks.

*When handling fresh chilies, wash hands immediately with hot soapy water and avoid touching face or eyes.

4: DETOXIFICATION DIET
Purging out your Bodily Poisons

Nutritional detoxification is the cornerstone of nutritional healing. When most people see the word detoxification, they usually think about clearing out the toxins in their body. For some, fasting comes to mind. And for good reason. The truth is that nutritional detoxification is the ongoing biochemical process of purging out destructive mind or matter from your body. Yes, it truly cleans the poisons out and, furthermore, keeps them out.

The Purging Detox Diet draws out the toxins. Detox works because it purges the darkness with suction-like efficiency out of its misery in hiding. The more effectively you purge, the deeper you dig down to the roots of your own personalized toxemia. Purging, as you know, leads to purification. The deeper you purge, the purer you get. And the better you feel. Also, the more you purge, the closer you get to the source of your ever-powerful healing heart and soul.

Purging nutritional detox gives your cellular dysfunctions a welcome chance to heal and get well. You see, the Hi·Lite Detox Diet takes your nutritional program right to the nucleus of the cell, where the Light of the soul is burning. And, as only penetrating detox can do, it fires up the Light in your cells. It then pumps up your blood and cleverly touches your cells with Hi·Lite hi-enzyme nutrients. This gently strokes your tissues in the right direction.

Nutritional detox is the turning point in your nutritional healing progress to balance the chemistry of your body. The net effect of detox is to favorably alter the acid-base balance of your tissues and body fluids. Detox naturally changes the chemistry of your body. It makes you more alkaline. Its hi-fiber cutting edge eliminates the sludge of your small intestine. This is why nutritional detox is fundamental to assuring complete assimilation. The high-quality food nutrients you eat need to be absorbed and effectively utilized before you can be optimally nourished. Detox makes this happen.

Before starting the diet, consult the Physiology and the Hi·Lights of Nutritional Detoxification.

<table>
<tr><td colspan="3" align="center">PHYSIOLOGY OF THE 7·DAY
NUTRITIONAL DETOXIFICATION DIET</td></tr>
<tr><td>DAY 8</td><td>PURGE·IT·OUT</td><td>CLEAR IT UP</td></tr>
<tr><td>DAY 9</td><td>EXPEL·IT·OUT</td><td>CAST IT OUT AND
ELIMINATE IT</td></tr>
<tr><td>DAY 10</td><td>BUST·IT·OUT</td><td>FIRE IT UP</td></tr>
<tr><td>DAY 11</td><td>TRANS·CEND·IT·THROUGH</td><td>SHIFT IT OVER</td></tr>
<tr><td>DAY 12</td><td>TRANS·CHANGE·IT·OVER</td><td>TAKE IT OVER</td></tr>
<tr><td>DAY 13</td><td>LEVEL·IT·OFF</td><td>KEEP UP WITH THE
BEAT</td></tr>
<tr><td>DAY 14</td><td>TRANS·FORM·IT</td><td>SHARPEN IT UP</td></tr>
</table>

The detoxification diet plan is essentially a natural vaccine. It is intended to stimulate your body's natural healing abilities to neutralize bodily impurities. Detox converts poisons into a form that is then ready to be excreted. The diet is prescribed to literally detoxify your body—to activate your bodily poisons, purify your bodily fluids, and remove harmful toxins from your cells. The result of effective detoxification is to increase your immunity.

Protection and prevention is the everyday business of a wholesome and sound, highly competent immune system. Your body's ability to detoxify the poisons in the air you breathe, the water you drink, and the food you eat is fundamental to your well-being. Your ability to weaken the impact of toxins is part and parcel of your detox plan. By lighting up your detox organs, your immunity shifts into high gear.

DAY 8: PURGE·IT·OUT

Detoxification *purges* excess mucus from your lymph and digestive systems. It also purges the phlegm from your lungs, the sludge from your bowels, the salt from your sweat, and the garbage from your liver, kidneys, and intestines. Mucus-like impurities that lie in the respiratory tract are cleared out, and mucilaginous impurities adherent to the intestinal tract will also be eliminated. The full evacuation of the poisons extracted is required to move the purging process along. Actually here's what happens.

DAY 9: EXPEL · IT · OUT

After one week on the Cleansing Diet, and a full day of juice fasting (the first day of your nutritional detox), the cells of the liver bed will get the message from the toxins circulating in the blood stream. It is time to fight back. Neutralize the poisons. Track them down. Fire away with toxicidal chemical soldiers. Interfere with what they are doing and wipe them out. And totally *eliminate* them from your body.

DAY 10: BUST · IT · OUT

The liver is your main organ of detoxification. The kidneys and the spleen also have detoxification potential. The pointed flame in the positive nutritional chemistry of the detox diet *fires up* these organs. In fact, it arouses the intuitive detoxifying powers of the liver, the spleen, and the kidneys.

Detoxification, therefore, calls for a high-level functioning of the liver, kidneys, and spleen. By Day 10, the diet sees to it that these organs are well cared for. It also means that top-notch structural and functional integrity of the organs of elimination—the colon, the lungs, the skin, and the kidneys—is needed to keep the detoxification machinery rolling.

DAY 11: TRANS · CEND · IT · THROUGH

Day 11 is pivotal to the detox process. It creates a smooth shift from just basic purging over to enhancing your immunological competence to heal and prevent disease. This continues as long as you follow the Hi·Lite dietary plan.

DAY 12: TRANS · CHANGE · IT · OVER

The net effect of detox is to line up a strong defense. And to recruit a courageous offense in the Light of a well-fed body chemistry. This is the wonder of nutritional detoxification. The combination of a strong offensive and defensive squad takes over your body chemistry.

DAY 13: LEVEL · IT · OFF

Staying in step with the detox process, you will get the job done. You don't have to move too quickly, and certainly your reflexes need to be quick so that you don't go too slowly. By keeping up with the beat of the detox, you begin to level off to a more optimal level of health and nourishment.

DAY 14: TRANSFORM·IT

Detoxification is the microscopic nutritional bridge between tox-emia and wellness. Your Hi·Lite Detox Diet is your all-star transfor-mation. The physiologic transmutation brings on a much higher level of resistance and greater level of well-being. In essence, then, nutritional detoxification sharpens up the process of purging, purification, and trans·mutation.

HI·ENZYME NUTRITIONAL DETOXIFICATION

Fresh fruits, raw vegetables, fruit juices, and raw vegetable juices, as well as sprouts, form the raw food backbone to the Detox Diet. In fact, the Detoxification Diet is predominantly a hi-enzyme, alkaline raw-food cleansing diet with the following modifications:

• **Higher fiber content.** The expansion of the basic Cleansing Diet into a Detox Diet relies on the input from whole grain cereals at breakfast, whole grain breads at lunch, and selected whole grains and/or legumes at dinner. The high fiber grains are rich in car-bohydrates, moderate in protein, and low in fat. The mechanical clout from the fiber adds substance to your diet. The high roughage in this program aids and abets the elimination of toxic wastes from the bile ducts to the intestines.

• **Higher protein intake.** The addition of whole grains as well as tofu, lima beans, and lentils provide a rich source of high-quality vegetable protein. It is interesting to note that much of this addi-tional protein, such as the tofu and lima beans, as well as millet and buckwheat, contribute to the high alkaline personality of this diet. Alkaline protein is a very special brand of natural ingredients. The Detox Diet is, therefore, a low-fat, high fiber, high natural car-bohydrate diet with a greater emphasis on vegetable protein. It is essentially a 1500 to 1800 calorie diet, with anywhere from 20 to 30 gms. of complete protein each day. The variety of essential amino acids added to the detox program enrich the liver and the kidneys, as well as the white and red blood corpuscles. They serve to strengthen the overall immunity of your system.

• **Magic potions for purging, healing, and transformation.** The hi-enzyme value of specialized nutritional supplements com-prise a vital dimension to the Detox Diet. Selected highly nutritious food items can enhance the therapeutic effectiveness of your detox program. These high-energy nutrients have the power to turn on the Light in the cells in your bone marrow, liver, kidneys, and spleen. These organs have the responsibility for your immunological com-petence and your ability to resist illness.

  • **BREWER'S YEAST** - a potent source of essential amino acids; also serves as a tonic to the liver.

- **BEE POLLEN** - a miracle food to build up your resistance.

- **RICE BRAN SYRUP** - a concentrated rich supply of B3 and other B complex vitamins.

- **WHEATGRASS JUICE** - abundant in chlorophyll, life force, and enzymes for total body nourishment.

- **SPIRULINA** - a blue-green microscopic algae, considered nature's most potent protein.

- **GINSENG** - an oriental wonder herb.

Brewer's yeast, bee pollen, and rice bran syrup blend well with fresh fruit and fresh fruit juices. This "Detox Smoothie" serves as a catalyst to the detox process taking place in the liver. Spirulina and wheatgrass juice are high chlorophyll nutrients that accelerate detoxification. Ginseng builds a strong body and nourishes your heart. It also strengthens your nerves and enhances your immunity. Ginseng is a marvelous addition to the detox diet. Don Quai is recommended instead of ginseng for females. These above supplements are an important nutritional tool to enhance the detox process. Mix your magic potions and match your makeup with more Energy from the Universe.

- **Juice fasting.** Juice fasting is an integral component of the Hi·Lite Detox Diet. In fact, it is an essential beginning to your week of detoxification. Juice fasting is known to accelerate and enhance the detoxifying power of liver, kidneys, and spleen. A one-day juice fast of fresh living juices, homemade potassium (broccoli-zuchini) vegetable broth, and detoxifying herbal teas is your burning bridge over the troubled toxic waters of your bodily fluids.

Juice fasting is one of the most fundamental tools of the Hi·Lite dietary program. Knowing how to juice fast is one of the most important skills of the health expert. Juice fasting eneables you to switch gears in a hurry and change direction. You see, juice fasting is a catalyst of the body's own inherent detoxification process. By allowing your digestive organs, liver, and kidneys to take a vacation, they can spend their time cleansing instead of digesting and metabolizing. When your body is preoccupied with eating and assimilating food, it leaves little time for the liver and kidneys to do anything else. Juice fasting, particularly after a cleansing diet has been initiated, and on a regular basis, flushes out your poisons. This is very basic to keeping your detox process going.

Regular one-day-per-week juice fasting is a vital dimension to your well-being. A one-day juice fast is a safe and reliable procedure. It will begin to relax your body's metabolic machinery, and give you a chance to regroup your healing efforts. At the same time, juice fasting will turn on the natural immune detox mechanisms.

For further information about fasting, Fast First. Then tune into your cosmic radio broadcast and refer to the final chapter in this book, "The Del Mar Diet **Permanent Weight Loss Program.**"

•**Higher B vitamin intake.** The additional supply of whole grains, magic potions, and high energy nutritional supplements provide a greater supply of essential B vitamins. This will enhance and aid your ability to totally assimilate the food you eat.

• *Nutritional supplements for the Detox Diet.*

VITAMIN B1	100 mg. twice a day (at breakfast and at dinner)
VITAMIN B6	200 mg. twice a day (at breakfast and at dinner)
HI-POTENCY B-COMPLEX (Super B or Mega B)	One with each meal as per the Cleansing Diet. (Contains a minimum of 50 mg. B_1, 50 mg. B_2, and 50 mg. B_3)
VITAMIN C	2500 mg. twice a day (at breakfast and at dinner)
MAGNESIUM OXIDE	250 mg. once a day
CHELATED ZINC	50 mg. once a day
VITAMIN E (Mixed Tocopherols)	400 I.U. 15 minutes before breakfast and 15 minutes before dinner

---

Hi·Lights of the Nutritional Detoxification Diet

The Hi·Lights of Nutritional Detox will light your way to understanding and successfully following the diet.

HI · LIGHTS OF NUTRITIONAL DETOXIFICATION — I:
BLUEPRINT FOR THE DETOXIFICATION DIET

Morning	Good Morning! 15-20 minutes of aerobics, deep breathing, and water initiation followed by:

Cosmic Interlude:	**THE DETOXIFICATION BREAKFAST** (7:00 — 8:00 a.m.)
	(1) Fresh seasonal fruit juice (6 oz.)
	    15 minutes later:
	(2) HI · LITE FRUIT SALAD SUPREME
	    with 2-3 fresh seasonal fruits, alfalfa sprouts (optional)
	(3) Almonds (5-6) or almond-sesame milk (3 oz.) with *1* of the following:
	    • High-fiber, crunchy granola, 2 oz.
	    • Whole grain cereal, 1 bowl

Mid-Morning:	**HI · LITE LIVER DETOXIFICATION SMOOTHY** (10:30 a.m.)
	Seasonal fruit juice, 6-8 oz., or 1 cup of seasonal fruit blended with
	    • 1½ Tbsp. brewers yeast
	    • 1 tsp. bee pollen
	    • 1 Tbsp. rice bran syrup

Mid-Afternoon	Sunshine; recharge your mind and body, followed by: **THE DETOXIFICATION LUNCHEON** (12:30 — 2:00 p.m.)

Cosmic Interlude:	(1) Fresh carrot juice (6 oz.)
	    15 minutes later:
	(2) HI · LITE LEAFY-GREEN CHLOROPHYLL SALAD
	    with your choice of HERBAL SALAD DRESSING and 1 of the following:
	    • 2 tsp. sesame seeds, or
	    • 1 stalk celery with 1-2 Tbsp. sesame-tahini nut butter
	(3) Whole grain breads, 1-2 slices to be chosen from:
	    • Sprouted wheat bread • Chapatis
	    • Sprouted 7-grain bread • Corn tortillas
	    • Whole wheat-sesame pita bread

Late Afternoon:	**SPECIALIZED DETOXIFICATION POTION** (3:30 p.m.)
	Your choice of *1* of the following:
	    • Carrot juice, 8 oz., with 1 tsp. Spirulina*
	    • Wheatgrass juice, 2 oz.

Evening	15 minutes of relaxation, followed by: **THE DETOXIFICATION VEGETARIAN DINNER** (5:30 — 7:00 p.m.)

Cosmic Interlude:	(1) Fresh carrot, carrot-celery, or carrot-celery-beet juice (8 oz.)
	    15 minutes later:
	(2) HI · LITE SPROUTED GARDEN-FRESH SALAD
	    with your choice of HERBAL SALAD DRESSING
	(3) STEAMED GREEN VEGETABLE COMBINATION
	    (a platter of 2-3 steamed green vegetables) or
	    BROCCOLI-MIXED GREENS VEGETABLE SOUP (1 bowl)
	(4) SELECTED COOKED WHOLE GRAINS OR LEGUMES, to be chosen from:
	    • Brown rice, ½ cup, with 2 tsp. sunflower seeds in salad
	    • Millet, ½ cup, with 2 tsp. sunflower seeds in salad
	    • Barley, ½ cup with 2 tsp. sunflower seeds in salad
	    • Tofu, 4 oz., with mushrooms, 4-8 medium, by itself or added to one of the above three dinner choices
	    • Peanut soup, 1 bowl
	    • Lentil soup, 1 bowl
	    • Lima bean-mixed vegetable soup, 1 bowl

*Special high-protein food supplement.

GUIDELINES FOR THE DETOXIFICATION DIET
FOODS EMPHASIZED ON THE DETOXIFICATION DIET

Seasonal Fresh Fruits and Fruit Juices	yes	All fresh fruits in season. FRESH FRUIT SALAD SUPREME limited to breakfast. Follow fruit precautions on Cleansing Diet. Emphasize watermelon, pear, orange, papaya.
Fresh Vegetables and Raw Vegetable Juices	yes	All fresh vegetables with an emphasis on carrots, beets, red onions, tomatoes, as well as leafy greens and steamed asparagus. 2 GARDEN-FRESH RAW SALADS daily. Follow vegetable precautions on Cleansing Diet.
Sprouts	yes	Living sprouts are essential to the Detoxification Diet. Emphasize alfalfa, bean, and sunflower seed sprouts.
Nuts	yes	Almonds can be added to granola or whole grain cereal for breakfast. Avoid all other nuts.
Nut Butter	yes	Sesame-tahini butter is the nut butter of choice. Avoid all other nut butters.
Seeds	yes	Sesame seeds or tahini for lunch, sunflower seeds for dinner when having cooked grains.
Natural Starchy Carbohydrates	no	On vacation. Not needed on Detoxification Diet.
Whole Grains	yes	Whole-grain cereals at breakfast, whole-grain breads at lunch, selected whole grains at dinner. Avoid all refined, processed breads, cereals, rice. Avoid all sugar in cereals and avoid eggs and sugar in bread. Avoid dextrose, table sugar, brown sugar, raw sugar, filtered honey, date sugar, jams, and syrupy spreads.
Legumes	yes	Choose from lentils, tofu, lima beans, or peanut soup for your dinner meal. Avoid other dried beans and peas on the Detoxification Diet.
Beverages	yes	One fresh raw seasonal fruit juice and two fresh raw vegetable juices daily. Follow precautions on Cleansing Diet. Mineral water with lime or bottled spring water to make herbal teas round out your fluid requirements. Add two specialized magic detoxification potions, one at 10:30 a.m. and another at 3:30 p.m.
Herbs	yes	Comfrey, dandelion, and white oak bark made into herbal teas. Ginseng highly recommended.
Seasonings	yes	The all-purpose herbs and condiments of the Cleansing Diet and the 7 basic herbs with an emphasis on lemon and garlic.
Dairy Products Milk, cheese Low-fat dairy Low-fat yogurt	no	All whole milk, cream, butter, eggs, margarine, low-fat milk products, sour cream, cheese, and dairy substitutes are excluded.
Flesh foods, meat, poultry, fish	no	Avoid; no exception, no cheating. Too heavy.

The bottom line is:
- 1 Fresh fruit salad daily.
- 2 Fresh leafy-green chlorophyll salads daily.
- 1 serving selected whole grains at each meal (legumes are acceptable at dinner).

- 1 steamed green vegetable or soup at dinner.
- 2 glasses carrot juice.
- 1 glass fruit juice.

HI·LIGHTS OF NUTRITIONAL DETOXIFICATION — III:
FOOD GROUPINGS FOR THE DETOXIFICATION DIET

When the proper food ingredients on the Dexotification Diet are combined together appropriately with respect to the laws of food combining, and with the purpose of establishing a detoxification regime, eight fundamental food groups exist.

GROUP 1:   **HI·LITE FRUIT SALAD SUPREMES**
The **FRUIT SALAD SUPREME** choices are the same as for Cleansing.

GROUP 1a: **FRESH FRUIT JUICES**
The fruit juice choices are the same as for the Cleansing Diet.

GROUP 2:   **HI·LITE CRISP LEAFY GREEN CHLOROPHYLL SALADS**
Refer to the Cleansing Diet. These groups remain the same with the following addition:

(1) **TABOULI SALAD.**

GROUP 2a: **FRESH RAW VEGETABLE JUICES**
The vegetable juice choices are the same as for the Cleansing Diet. Carrot or carrot-celery-beet is preferred.

GROUP 3:   **STEAMED GREEN VEGETABLE COMBINATIONS**
The steamed vegetable combinations are the same as for Cleansing.

GROUP 4:   **SELECTED WHOLE GRAIN CEREALS**
Add 5-6 almonds or 3 oz. almond-sesame milk to one of the following:

(1) **SHARON'S CRUNCHY GRANOLA**   (4) Cooked seven-grain cereals
(2) **CINNAMON-OAT CEREAL**   (5) Cooked millet
(3) Bran-granola, oil free   (6) Cream of rye or cream of wheat

GROUP 5:   **SELECTED WHOLE GRAIN BREADS**

(1) Sprouted wheat bread   (4) Chapatis
(2) Sprouted 7-grain bread   (5) Corn tortillas
(3) Whole wheat-sesame pita bread

GROUP 6:   **SELECTED COOKED WHOLE GRAINS**
When choosing one of the following, add 2 tsp. sunflower seeds to dinner salad, and mix in (optional) 2-3 oz. of tofu:

(1) Brown rice   (3) Barley   (5) Buckwheat
(2) Wild rice   (4) Millet

GROUP 7:   **SELECTED LEGUMES**

(1) Tofu (high-protein soy curd) (2-4 oz. can be added to selected whole grains)
(2) Lentils
(3) Peanut soup
(4) Lima bean-vegetable soup

GROUP 8:   **HERBAL SALAD DRESSINGS**
The herbal salad dressings are the same as for the Cleansing Diet with the following addition:

(1) **SESAME-TAHINI DRESSING** (tahini, lemon, garlic, kelp, dill). This can be used on the luncheon salad. Omit sesame seeds in salad.

HI·LIGHTS OF NUTRITIONAL DETOXIFICATION — IV:
GOLDEN RULES FOR THE DETOXIFICATION DIET

Follow these simple rules to get the most out of your Detoxification program:

RULE NO. 1: • **EAT THREE MEALS A DAY.**

RULE NO. 2: • **BREAKFAST BETWEEN 7:00 to 8:00 a.m. FOR 30 MINUTES.**
- Drink 1 glass (6 oz.) of **fresh fruit juice** from the corresponding season in **Group 1a.** *15 minutes later:*
- Select 1 **FRUIT SALAD SUPREME** from **Group 1** in accordance with the appropriate season.
- Add 1 **SELECTED WHOLE GRAIN CEREAL** from **Group 4.**

RULE NO. 3: • **MIDWAY BETWEEN BREAKFAST AND LUNCH (approximately 10:30 a.m.) DRINK LIVER DETOXIFICATION SMOOTHY.**

RULE NO. 4: • **LUNCH BETWEEN 12:30 to 2:00 p.m. FOR 30 MINUTES.**
- Drink 6 oz. of fresh carrot juice.
- Select 1 **LEAFY-GREEN CHLOROPHYLL SALAD** from **Group 2.**
- Add 2 tsp. sesame seeds to the salad or 1 tbsp. tahini butter on celery or 2 tbsp. **TAHINI SALAD DRESSING.**
- Choose 1 **HERBAL SALAD DRESSING** from **Group 8.**
- Select 1-2 slices **WHOLE GRAIN BREAD** from **Group 5.**

RULE NO. 5: • **MIDWAY BETWEEN LUNCH AND DINNER (approximately 3:30 p.m.) DRINK SPECIALIZED DETOXIFICATION POTION.** (1 tsp. Spirulina in 6-8 oz. carrot juice or 2 oz. wheatgrass juice)

RULE NO. 6: • **DINE BETWEEN 5:00 to 7:00 p.m. ALLOW AT LEAST 30 MINUTES AND UP TO 90 MINUTES FOR A PLEASANT, ENJOYABLE DINNER.**
- Drink 8 oz. of fresh carrot, fresh carrot-celery, or fresh carrot-celery-beet juice 15 minutes before your main vegetarian dinner.
- Select 1 **LEAFY-GREEN CHLOROPHYLL SALAD** from **Group 2.**
- Choose 1 **HERBAL SALAD DRESSING** from **Group 8.**
- Select 1 **STEAMED GREEN VEGETABLE COMBINATION** from **Group 3.**
- Add 1 serving of **COOKED WHOLE GRAINS** from **Group 6** with 2 tsp. sunflower seeds added to salad OR select 1 **PROTEINACEOUS LEGUME** from **Group 7.**

RULE NO. 7: • **AVOID SNACKING.**

RULE NO. 8: • **AVOID DAIRY PRODUCTS OR FLESH PROTEIN.**

RULE NO. 9: • **TAKE AT LEAST 30 MINUTES TO ENJOY EACH MEAL.**

RULE NO. 10: • **RELAX WITH YOUR MEALS. CHEW EACH BITE SLOWLY.**

RULE NO. 11: • **DRINK DETOXIFICATION HERBAL REMEDY FROM WHITE OAK BARK-COMFREY — AND DANDELION ROOT BETWEEN YOUR MEALS.** You can add some peppermint to this tea, as well. Emphasize Ginseng for men and Don Quai for women. Be certain to drink 6-8 glasses of fluid each day.

RULE NO. 12: • **SEASON YOUR FOODS WITH THE HERBS AND CONDIMENTS FROM THE CLEANSING DIET WITH AN EMPHASIS ON GARLIC.**

RULE NO. 13: • **EMPHASIZE BEETS, LEMONS, AND PAPAYAS IN THE DETOXIFICATION DIET.**

RULE NO. 14: • **USE SESAME-TAHINI BUTTER INSTEAD OF PEANUT BUTTER, ALMOND BUTTER, OR CASHEW BUTTER ON THE DETOXIFICATION DIET.**

JUICE FASTING

(1) Select 6-8 oz. **fresh fruit juice**, alternating every three hours with **fresh vegetable juice**. Choose the fresh fruit juices from the corresponding season. Fresh carrot juice, carrot-celery juice, or carrot-celery-beet juice can serve for all seasons.

(2) Drink herbal teas as desired. Listen to your body.

(3) Prepare a highly alkaline, potassium-rich vegetable broth for evenings, cold afternoons, winter or rainy days to supplement your fresh juices and herbal remedies. Drink the following vegetable broth as desired:

Zucchini, 1 cup	Carrot, 1 medium
Broccoli, ½ cup	Potato, 1 medium
String beans, ½ cup	Celery, 1 stalk
Parsley, 1 Tbsp.	Beet, 1 medium

Add the above vegetables to 4 cups boiling water and let it simmer for 20 minutes. Discard vegetables and drink the broth. Season with garlic, onion, cayenne, and kelp.

JUICE FAST SCHEDULE

Spring:
7:00 a.m. —	orange or watermelon
10:00 a.m. —	carrot
1:00 p.m. —	orange or watermelon
4:00 p.m. —	carrot
7:00 p.m. —	orange or watermelon
10:00 p.m. —	carrot-celery or carrot-celery-beet

Summer:
7:00 a.m. —	watermelon
10:00 a.m. —	carrot
1:00 p.m. —	watermelon
4:00 p.m. —	carrot
7:00 p.m. —	watermelon
10:00 p.m. —	carrot-celery or carrot-celery-beet

Autumn: *
7:00 a.m. —	apple
10:00 a.m. —	carrot
1:00 p.m. —	apple
4:00 p.m. —	carrot
7:00 p.m. —	apple
10:00 p.m. —	carrot-celery or carrot-celery-beet

Winter:
7:00 a.m. —	orange or grapefruit or pineapple
10:00 a.m. —	carrot
1:00 p.m. —	orange or grapefruit or pineapple
4:00 p.m. —	carrot
7:00 p.m. —	orange or grapefruit or pineapple
10:00 p.m. —	carrot-celery or carrot-celery-beet

One hour for introspection and verbal fasting, preferably early in the morning, is highly recommended.

---

* Carrot-apple is an acceptable combination for autumn juice fast.

HI·LITE NUTRITIONAL DETOXIFICATION BREAKFAST
(7:00-8:00 a.m.)

Spring:
(1) Papaya-pineapple juice (6 oz.)
    15 minutes later
(2) **SOUTH AMERICAN TROPICAL FRUIT SALAD**
   • Papaya, ½ cup
   • Pineapple, ½ cup
   • Banana, 1 medium
(3) **SHARON'S CRUNCHY GRANOLA** (2 oz.), with
   • Almonds, 5-6 or almond-sesame milk, 3 oz.)
   Alfalfa sprouts (optional)

Summer:
(1) Watermelon juice (6 oz.)
    15 minutes later
(2) **SUMMER MELON SALAD**
   • Canteloupe, ½ medium
   • Watermelon, ½ cup
   • Honeydew, ½ cup
(3) **SHARON'S CRUNCHY GRANOLA** (2 oz.), with
   • Almonds, 5-6 or almond-sesame milk, 3 oz.
   Alfalfa sprouts (optional)

Autumn:
(1) Apple juice (6 oz.) *15 minutes later*
(2) **WALDORF APPLE SALAD AMBROSIA**
   • Pippin apple, ½ medium
   • Pear, ½ medium
   • Banana, 1 medium
(3) **SHARON'S CRUNCHY GRANOLA** (2 oz.), with
   • Almonds, 5-6 or almond-sesame milk, 3 oz.
   Alfalfa sprouts (optional)

Winter:
(1) Orange juice (6 oz.) *15 minutes later*
(2) **WINTER CITRUS SALAD**
   • Orange, 1 medium
   • Pink grapefruit, ½ medium
   • Pineapple, ½ cup
(2) **SHARON'S CRUNCHY GRANOLA** (2 oz.), with
   • Almonds, 5-6 or almond-sesame milk, 3 oz.
   Alfalfa sprouts (optional)

HI·LITE NUTRITIONAL DETOXIFICATION LUNCHEON
(12:30-2:00 p.m.)

(1) Fresh carrot or carrot-celery-beet juice (6 oz.) *15 minutes later*
(2) **SUPER SPROUT SALAD**
   • Bean sprouts, all you want
   • Alfalfa sprouts, all you want
   • Sunflower seed sprouts, all you want
   • Romaine lettuce, 4 leaves
   • Tomato, ½ large
   • Red onion, ¼ cup
   • Sesame seeds, 2 tsp.
      • HERBAL VINAIGRETTE DRESSING
(3) Sprouted seven-grain bread, 1-2 slices.

HI·LITE NUTRITIONAL DETOXIFICATION DINNER
(5:30-7:00 p.m.)

(1) Fresh carrot juice (8 oz.) *15 minutes later*
(2) **GARDEN-GREEN CHLOROPHYLL SALAD**
   • Romaine lettuce, 2-4 leaves
   • Spinach, 4 leaves
   • Alfalfa sprouts, ½ cup
   • Tomato, ½ large
   • Swiss chard, 1-2 leaves
   • Parsley, 1 Tbsp.
   • Red onion, ¼ medium
   • Carrot, 1 medium
      • KELP-FROM-THE-SEA DRESSING
(3) BROCCOLI-MIXED GREENS VEGETABLE SOUP
(4) ZUCCHINI-RICE CASSEROLE
   • Zucchini, ½ cup
   • String beans, ½ cup
   • Brown rice, ½ cup

HI·LITE NUTRITIONAL DETOXIFICATION BREAKFAST
(7:00-8:00 a.m.)

Spring:
(1) Orange juice (6 oz.)
  15 minutes later
(2) **ZESTY SPRING SALAD**
  • Pineapple, ½ cup
  • Banana, 1 medium
  • Strawberries, 5 large
(3) Seven-grain cereal, 1 bowl, with almonds, 5-6 or almond-sesame milk, 3 oz.
  Alfalfa sprouts (optional)

Summer:
(1) Watermelon juice (6 oz.)
  15 minutes later
(2) **SUMMER MELON SALAD**
  • Cantaloupe, ½ medium
  • Watermelon, ½ cup
  • Honeydew, ½ cup
(3) Seven-grain cereal, 1 bowl with almonds, 5-6 or almond-sesame milk, 3 oz.
  Alfalfa sprouts (optional)

Autumn:
(1) Pear juice (6 oz.) *15 minutes later*
(2) **MIXED APPLE SALAD**
  • Pippin apple, ½ medium
  • MacIntosh apple, ½ medium
  • Golden Delicious apple, ½ med.
(3) Seven-grain cereal, 1 bowl, with almonds, 5-6 or almond-sesame milk, 3 oz.
  Alfalfa sprouts (as many as you want)

Winter:
(1) Orange juice (6 oz.) *15 minutes later*
(2) **ORANGE WONDERLAND SALAD**
  • Orange, ½ medium
  • Pineapple, ½ cup
  • Banana, ½ medium
(3) Seven-grain cereal, 1 bowl, with almonds, 5-6 or almond-sesame milk, 3 oz.
  Alfalfa sprouts (as many as you want)

HI·LITE NUTRITIONAL DETOXIFICATION LUNCHEON
(12:30-2:00 p.m.)

(1) Fresh carrot-celery-beet juice (6 oz.) *15 minutes later*

(2) **TABOULI SALAD**
  • Romaine lettuce, 4 leaves
  • Alfalfa sprouts, ½ cup
  • Tomato, ½ large
  • Bulgar wheat, ½ cup cooked
  • Celery, stalk
  • Cucumber, six ½ inch slices
  • Green pepper, ¼ large
  • LEMON-TAHINI DRESSING
(3) Pita whole-wheat sesame bread; you may cut pita bread open, fill with Tabouli salad, and eat in the form of a vegetable sandwich.

HI·LITE NUTRITIONAL DETOXIFICATION DINNER
(5:30-7:00 p.m.)

(1) Fresh carrot juice (6-8 oz.) *15 minutes later*
(2) **GARDEN-GREEN CHLOROPHYLL SALAD**
  • Romaine lettuce, 2-4 leaves
  • Spinach, 4 leaves
  • Alfalfa sprouts, ½ cup
  • Tomato, ½ large
  • Swiss chard, 1-2 leaves
  • Parsley, 1 Tbsp.
  • Red onion, ¼ medium
  • Carrot, 1 medium
  • LEMON-GARLIC DRESSING
(3) VEGETABLE CHOP SUEY
  • Steamed selected Chinese greens (bok-choy, Chinese peas, mung bean sprouts)
  • Tofu, 4 oz.
  • ½ cup brown rice.

HI · LITE NUTRITIONAL DETOXIFICATION BREAKFAST
(7:00-8:00 a.m.)

Spring:
(1) Papaya juice (6 oz.)
15 minutes later
(2) **MANGO DAYBREAK DELIGHT**
- Mango, ½ medium
- Banana, ½ medium
- Pineapple, ½ cup
(3) Bran granola (2 oz.) with almonds, 5-6 or almond-sesame milk, 3 oz. Alfalfa sprouts (as many as you want)

Summer:
(1) Papaya juice (6 oz.)
15 minutes later
(2) **CHERRY-FRIAR PLUM SALAD**
- Cherries, 8
- Friar plum, 1
- Nectarine, 1 medium
(3) Bran granola (2 oz.) with almonds, 5-6 or almond-sesame milk, 3 oz. Alfalfa sprouts (as many as you want)

Autumn:
(1) Apple juice (6 oz.)
15 minutes later
(2) **AUTUMN ENERGY SALAD**
- Pippin apple, ½ medium
- Papaya, ½ cup
- Banana, 1 medium
(3) Bran granola (2 oz.) with almonds, 5-6 or almond-sesame milk, 3 oz. Alfalfa sprouts (as many as you want)

Winter:
(1) Grapefruit juice (6 oz.)
15 minutes later
(2) **PAPAYA PARADISE SALAD**
- Orange, ½ medium
- Papaya, ½ cup
- Banana, 1 medium
(3) Bran granola (2 oz.) with almonds, 5-6 or almond-sesame milk, 3 oz. Alfalfa sprouts (as many as you want)

HI · LITE NUTRITIONAL DETOXIFICATION LUNCHEON
(12:30-2:00 p.m.)

(1) Fresh carrot-celery-beet juice (6-8 oz.)
15 minutes later
(2) **RADIANT RADISH SALAD**
- Romaine lettuce, 4 leaves
- Alfalfa sprouts, ½ cup
- Tomato, ½ large
- Radishes, 2 small
- Red onion, ¼ cup
- Chopped parsley, 1 Tbsp.
  - **HERBAL ITALIAN DRESSING**
  - Sesame seeds, 2 tsp.
(3) MELTZER B.L.T. SANDWICH (bread, lettuce, tomato): 2 slices toasted sprouted 7-grain bread made into a sandwich.

HI · LITE NUTRITIONAL DETOXIFICATION DINNER
(5:30-7:00 p.m.)

(1) Fresh carrot or carrot-celery-beet juice (8 oz.)
15 minutes later
(2) **JICAMA-BEET TREAT**
- Jicama
- Raw grated beet, ½ medium
- Carrot, 1 small
- Romaine lettuce, 4 leaves
- Tomato, ½ large
- Alfalfa sprouts, ½ cup
  - **KELP-FROM-THE-SEA DRESSING**
  - sunflower seeds, 2 tsp.
(3) MIXED GREENS VEGETABLE SOUP
(4) BROCCOLI-BROWN RICE CASSEROLE — with or without tofu

HI·LITE NUTRITIONAL DETOXIFICATION BREAKFAST
(7:00-8:00 a.m.)

Spring:
(1) Papaya juice (6 oz.)
   15 minutes later
(2) **GRAPE DELIGHT SALAD**
   • Seedless green grapes, 1 cup
   • Red grapes, ½ cup
   • Concord grapes, ½ cup
(3) Cooked millet, 1 bowl, with almonds,
   5-6 or almond-sesame milk, 3 oz.
   Alfalfa sprouts (optional)

Summer:
(1) Papaya juice (6 oz.)
   15 minutes later
(2) **HAWAIIAN FRUIT SALAD**
   • Papaya, ½ cup
   • Mango, ½ cup
   • Pineapple, ½ cup
(3) Cooked millet, 1 bowl, with
   almonds, 5-6 or almond-sesame
   milk, 3 oz.
   Alfalfa sprouts (optional)

Autumn:
(1) Apple juice (6 oz.)
   15 minutes later
(2) **PEACEFUL PEAR SALAD**
   • Pear, 1 medium
   • Papaya, 1 cup
   • Banana, 1 medium
(3) Cooked millet, 1 bowl, with almonds,
   5-6 or almond-sesame milk, 3 oz.
   Alfalfa sprouts (optional)

Winter:
(1) Orange juice (6 oz.)
   15 minutes later
(2) **PINK GRAPEFRUIT WINTER
   SALAD**
   • Pink grapefruit, ½ medium
   • Orange, ½ medium
   • Banana, 1 medium
(3) Cooked millet, 1 bowl, with
   almonds, 5-6 or almond-sesame
   milk, 3 oz.
   Alfalfa sprouts (optional)

HI·LITE NUTRITIONAL DETOXIFICATION LUNCHEON
(12:30-2:00 p.m.)

(1) Fresh carrot juice (6 oz.) *15 minutes later*
(2) **MEXICAN CABBAGE SALAD**
   • Red cabbage, ¼ cup
   • Green cabbage, ¼ cup
   • Red onion, ¼ cup
   • Romaine lettuce, 4 leaves
   • Alfalfa sprouts, ½ cup
   • Tomato, ½ large
       • LEMON-GARLIC DRESSING
         • 2 tsp. sesame seeds
(3) Corn tortillas, 1-2; fill tortillas with salad

HI·LITE NUTRITIONAL DETOXIFICATION DINNER
(5:30-7:00 p.m.)

(1) Fresh carrot or carrot-celery-beet juice (8 oz.) *15 minutes later*
(2) **SPICE-OF-LIFE SPINACH SALAD**
   • Spinach, 4 leaves
   • Romaine lettuce, 2-4 leaves
   • Tomato, ½ large
   • Alfalfa sprouts, ½ cup
   • Red onion, ¼ medium
   • Celery, 1 stalk
       • ITALIAN HERBAL DRESSING
         • sunflower seeds, 2 tsp.
(3) LENTIL-VEGETABLE CASSEROLE
   • Lentils
   • Broccoli
   • String beans
   • Cauliflower
       or LENTIL-VEGETABLE SOUP

HI · LITE NUTRITIONAL DETOXIFICATION BREAKFAST
(7:00-8:00 a.m.)

Spring:
(1) Pineapple juice (6 oz.)
    15 minutes later
(2) **ZESTY SPRING SALAD**
    • Pineapple, ½ cup
    • Banana, 1 medium
    • Strawberries, 5 large
(3) Almond crunch or bran granola
    (2 oz.) with almonds, 5-6 or
    almond-sesame milk, 3 oz.
    Alfalfa sprouts (as many as you
    want)

Summer:
(1) Papaya juice (6 oz.)
    15 minutes later
(2) **MANGO PEACH SALAD**
    • Mango, ½ medium
    • Peach, 1 medium
    • Banana, ½ medium
(3) Almond crunch or bran granola
    (2 oz.) with almonds, 5-6 or
    almond-sesame milk, 3 oz.
    Alfalfa sprouts (as many as you
    want)

Autumn:
(1) Pear juice (6 oz.)
    15 minutes later
(2) **WALDORF APPLE SALAD
    AMBROSIA**
    • Pippin apple, 1 medium
    • Pear, ½ medium
    • Banana, 1 medium
(3) Almond crunch or bran granola
    (2 oz.) with almonds, 5-6 or
    almond-sesame milk, 3 oz.
    Alfalfa sprouts (as many as you
    want)

Winter:
(1) Orange juice (6 oz.)
    15 minutes later
(2) **SOUTH AMERICAN TROPICAL
    FRUIT SALAD**
    • Pineapple, ½ cup
    • Papaya, ½ cup
    • Banana, 1 medium
(3) Almond crunch or bran granola
    (2 oz.) with almonds, 5-6 or
    almond-sesame milk, 3 oz.
    Alfalfa sprouts (as many as you
    want)

HI · LITE NUTRITIONAL DETOXIFICATION LUNCHEON
(12:30-2:00 p.m.)

(1) Fresh carrot or carrot-celery-beet juice (6 oz.) *15 minutes later*
(2) **GARDEN PEA SALAD**
    • Chinese snow peas, 12
    • Romaine lettuce, 4 leaves
    • Green peas, 2 Tbsp.
    • ONION-GARLIC DRESSING
    • Green pepper, ½ large
    • Alfalfa sprouts, ½ cup
    • Tomato, ½ large
    • Sesame or sunflower seeds, 2 tsp.
(3) Chapatis, 1-2 (which can be slightly heated). Place the vegetables inside the
    chapati for a sandwich.

HI · LITE NUTRITIONAL DETOXIFICATION DINNER
(5:30-7:00 p.m.)

(1) Fresh carrot or carrot-celery-beet juice (8 oz.) *15 minutes later*
(2) **RAW MUSHROOM SALAD**
    • Romaine lettuce, 4 leaves
    • Sprouts, ½ cup
    • Tomato, ½ large
    • Mushrooms, 10 small or 4 large
    • Cucumber, six 1/8 inch slices
    • Celery, 1 stalk
    • LEMON-VINAIGRETTE DRESSING
    • Sunflower seeds, 2 tsp.
(3) LIMA BEAN-MIXED VEGETABLE SOUP

HI·LITE NUTRITIONAL DETOXIFICATION BREAKFAST
(7:00-8:00 a.m.)

Spring:
(1) Orange juice (6 oz.)
    15 minutes later
(2) **SOUTH AMERICAN TROPICAL FRUIT SALAD**
   • Papaya, ½ cup
   • Banana, 1 medium
   • Pineapple, ½ cup
(3) **CINNAMON-OAT CEREAL**
   1 bowl, with almonds, 5-6, or almond-sesame milk, 3 oz.
   Alfalfa sprouts (optional)

Summer:
(1) Papaya juice (6 oz.)
    15 minutes later
(2) **NECTARINE-PEACH SALAD**
   • Nectarine, 1 medium
   • Peach, 1 medium
   • Cherries, 8
(3) **CINNAMON-OAT CEREAL**
   1 bowl, with almonds, 5-6, or almond-sesame milk, 3 oz.
   Alfalfa sprouts (optional)

Autumn:
(1) Apple juice (6 oz.)
    15 minutes later
(2) **AUTUMN ENERGY SALAD**
   • Pippin apple, ½ medium
   • Papaya, ½ cup
   • Banana, 1 medium
(3) **CINNAMON-OAT CEREAL**
   1 bowl with almonds, 5-6 or almond-sesame milk, 3 oz.
   Alfalfa sprouts (optional) want)

Winter:
(1) Orange juice (6 oz.)
    15 minutes later
(2) **PINK GRAPEFRUIT WINTER SALAD**
   • Pink grapefruit, ½ medium
   • Orange, ½ medium
   • Banana, 1 medium
(3) **CINNAMON-OAT CEREAL**
   1 bowl with almonds, 5-6 or almond-sesame milk, 3 oz.
   Alfalfa sprouts (optional)

HI·LITE NUTRITIONAL DETOXIFICATION LUNCHEON
(12:30-2:00 p.m.)

(1) Fresh carrot or carrot-celery-beet juice (8 oz.) *15 minutes later*

(2) **SPICE-OF-LIFE SPINACH SALAD**
   • Spinach, 4 leaves
   • Romaine lettuce, 2-4 leaves
   • Tomato, ½ large
        • ONION-GARLIC DRESSING
   • Alfalfa sprouts, ½ cup
   • Red onion, ¼ medium
   • Celery, 1 stalk
   • Sesame seeds, 2 tsp.
(3) Sprouted whole wheat bread, 1-2 slices

HI·LITE NUTRITIONAL DETOXIFICATION DINNER
(5:30-7:00 p.m.)

(1) Fresh carrot or carrot-celery-beet juice (8 oz.) *15 minutes later*

(2) **CUCUMBER-BEET SALAD**
   • Romaine lettuce, 4 leaves
   • Cucumber
   • Raw shredded beet, ½ medium
        • ITALIAN DRESSING
   • Tomato, ½ large
   • Alfalfa sprouts, ½ cup
   • Carrot, 1 small
(3) CAULIFLOWER MIXED VEGETABLE PLATTER
   • Zucchini, 1 cup
   • Cauliflower, ½ cup
   • Broccoli, ½ cup
(4) PEANUT SOUP or BROWN RICE WITH TOFU AND MUSHROOM CASSEROLE

DETOXIFY TO GET WELL

The benefit of the Detox Diet is the sense of well-being that comes from allowing your body to exist in a more positive biochemical state. This nutritional program focuses on sharpening your often-neglected immune system. Getting yourself a chance to clean up and sweep out the residue from the Cleansing Diet is an additional asset of the 7-day program. The high fiber mechanical clout of the Detox Diet eliminates unwanted toxins from the body. Once these toxins are efficiently expelled, mental and physical well-being, the natural healing state of human function, can be more readily restored.

The discipline of the Detox Diet is also an important meditation. It opens your mind to the joy of your emotions. The Detox Diet is one of the four wheels of your Hi·Lite nutritional program (cleansing, detox, maintenance, and juice fasting). It is usually prescribed as a 5-6 day mid-seasonal cleansing during the first two years of your wellness program. This means that the first week in November, the first week in February, the first week in May, and the first week in August are detox times. The diet is particularly indicated for individuals who suffer from liver dysfunction, poor assimilation, or nervous conditions. It is also a strategic diet for those with poor elimination. It serves as a more gentle cleansing for the elderly, senior citizens, or teenagers and children when cleansing is so advised. It often serves as the initial diet to kick off the regeneration of burned out degenerative nerve conditions such as is seen in patients with multiple sclerosis, strokes, and nutritional deficiency states.

DETOXIFICATION IS YOUR MAGIC CODE TO CLEAR OUT

The truth is that nutritional detoxification is one definitive factor that slows down the aging process. Detoxification preserves the physical dignity of the human body. In this way you will continue to look better, as well as feel young, with the passage of time.

Mary Ellen was an attractive, well-dressed, 56-year-old claims adjuster. She had red hair, a warm smile, and a loving personality. Ever since her most recent birthday, four months ago, she had found herself in an emotional turmoil.

"There is so much frustration and stress in my everyday life. Doctor, I'm on the verge of ending my relationship with my second husband. We've been married for fifteen years and have grown very attached to each other. My first marriage lasted a disappointing nine years. I seem to be shackled to my past and preoccupied with my future. To be perfectly candid, I'm afraid I will be all alone for the final years of my life. I feel as if my life is passing me by."

"What do you mean by that?"

Mary Ellen took a deep breath. "Well, my bones and my body do not feel alive the way they used to. I wake up in the morning and it takes me quite some time before the stiffness leaves my spine. Most of the time I don't even want to get out of bed."

"How do you feel once you get started?"

"At times good and at times not so hot. Some days my moods change so rapidly, I feel I'm out of control. I know something funny is happening to me."

"Why?"

"My memory isn't what it used to be. And I don't sleep well. A few weeks ago, I had the most horrifying experience of my life."

"What happened to you?"

"I suddenly awoke in the middle of the night. I suppose I was having a bad dream. I got up to eat some stew that was left over from the night before. I didn't get to the second helping before my chest began to ache. It felt like a constant pressure. Pins and needles started going down both my arms. I thought I was dying. I rushed over to the local emergency room."

"What did they find?"

"The doctor did an electrocardiogram, took a chest X-ray, and did all kinds of tests. They couldn't find anything wrong with me. They told me I was having an anxiety attach. They sent me to an internist."

"What did the internist say?"

"He told me I was as healthy as a horse and that I look as good for my age as he does. I told him I feel like an unwanted dried up prune. He prescribed valium and I know that's not good for my health. I don't want to take any tranquilizers. I've become a slave to my emotions. The psychiatrist they sent me to put me on anti-depressants. I don't want to see any more psychiatrists, and I'm not interested in taking any more drugs. I'm tired of these emotional ups and downs which, come to think of it, have been almost all down of late. There must be a more natural way that you can help me."

"I think so, Mary Ellen."

A complete physical and a battery of routine lab tests checked out normal. They did not provide any clue as to why Mary Ellen was in such a disorganized state.

"Tell me, what is your diet like?"

"I think I eat pretty well. Except maybe in the morning when I usually eat on the run. For breakfast I'll fix a couple of eggs. I usually have a glass of apple juice and some whole wheat toast. At lunch I grab something at the local seafood house. I usually order a tuna salad with hard-boiled eggs. Other days I'll have a cheeseburger or get a slice of pizza with some diet pepsi. For dinner I usually have beef, chicken, or fish with some garden vegetables. I snack on wheat thins, popcorn, or raisins when I get hungry. I know enough not to add any salt or sugar to my foods."

When I analysed Mary Ellen's diet, I determined that the amount of acid-forming foods she ate was anywhere from two to four times as much as the alkaline-forming foods she consumed. I calculated her dietary alkaline-to-acid ratio to be nearly 1:3. At times it ranged anywhere from 1:2 to 1:4.

OPTIMAL ALKALINE / ACID RATIO

The optimal alkaline to acid ratio to sustain excellent health ranges from 3:2 to 3:1 (not to go below 1:1) in accordance to your needs. Over-acidity, Mary Ellen's condition, or even a ratio of 1:1 acid-forming to alkaline-forming food, gram for gram, ounce per ounce in a diet contributes to subtle metabolic imbalances. This, in turn, is responsible for commonly undiagnosed hypersensitive food allergies. In addition, over-acidity constipates your emotions, hardens your mind, and stiffens your body. It poisons your body fluids and rusts your nerve endings. Over-acidity also wears away the integrity of your joints.

On the basis of her over-acid condition, Mary Ellen's body chemistry was anything but balanced. The lack of fresh fruits with her breakfast, the lack of fresh green leafy vegetables at lunch, and the emphasis on fish and eggs threw her dietary intake into a decidedly acid residue state. The over-acidity interfered with her body's ability to *assimilate* essential B-vitamins and needed complex carbohydrates. These two special nutrients, the B-vitamins and complex carbohydrates, are indispensable to the chemistry necessary for the brain and nervous system to function best.

In this fashion, Mary Ellen's diet had created a relative low-grade

B-vitamin deficiency. There just weren't enough B-complex vitamins and quality carbohydrates absorbed to nourish all the organs. And to add insult to injury, her high level of emotional stress more than doubled her B-vitamin requirements. Her nervous system paid the price. Her poor assimilation caused unnecessary chemical stress on the steadiness of her blood sugar, as well as setting her up for even more harmful food allergies. These bio-chemical imbalances laid the groundwork for her emotional disequilibrium. Her daily chaos landed on the infected nutritional soil that favored the growth of her emotional stress.

I explained to Mary Ellen that she needed to correct her nutritionally based B-vitamin and carbohydrate imbalances. I wanted her to appreciate that a well-balanced body chemistry has a *balancing effect* on the emotions. I was hoping she would understand that she could not expect her emotional life to come into balance when her body chemistry was out of balance.

"Mary Ellen, the time has come to detoxify your body. The high alkaline reserve of a detoxification program will correct your acid-alkaline imbalance. Detoxification literally means inactivating the acid poisons that have found their way into your body. These poisons gradually build up from years and years of improper eating habits. Once cleansing is initiated, these acidic toxins break loose from your cells and begin to move into your circulation. In the bloodstream they are buffered by the alkaline chemistry of your plasma. Then these poisons are carried to the detoxification burial grounds of the liver, the kidneys, and the spleen before they are eliminated. The circulating acid toxins are the physiological explanation for what some individuals describe as the tired, drugged, nauseating, or headachy feeling they may experience while they are "detoxifying" on a detoxification diet. In fact, one of the distinguishing features of a detoxification diet is its ability to restore the proper acid-alkaline body chemistry, and this is fundamental to establishing your optimal nutritional biochemical balance.

"You see, the proper ratio of alkaline-forming foods to acid-forming foods is vital to the optimal function of intracellular bodily enzymes. These include the all-important digestive enzymes as well as those in the liver and the rest of the body. That is why the proper alkaline to acid ratio is so essential to maintaining optimal health, increasing your resistance to disease, and in fact, preventing disease. A hi-enzyme, high alkaline diet feeds and lubricates your enzymatic machinery. This is basic to establishing nutritional biochemical balance. Most popular diets overlook this longevity secret."

"What do you mean by acid-forming and alkaline-forming?" Mary Ellen asked.

"All your foods are digested and burned, leaving either an alkaline ash, an acid ash, or a neutral ash. The mineral composition of the food determines which foods will be acid, neutral, or alkaline. Fresh vegetables and fresh fruits are rich in potassium and magnesium. They leave an alkaline ash after digestion. When more phosphorous, sulfur, or chlorine remains in the body than potassium or magnesium after the food has been burned or digested, the food will leave an acid ash. Oranges, lemons, grapefruits, and pineapples, and other fruits containing citric and malic acids have an acid or sour taste, but in fact actually yield a milder potassium alkaline ash after they are digested."

"How can I find out which foods are acid-forming and which are alkaline-forming?"

"I have a chart (see below) you can take home with you to give you an overview. Remember that *fresh leafy green vegetables, fresh fruits, almonds, soybeans, lima beans, and selected whole grains, in particular, buckwheat and millet, are alkaline forming. These are staples to your Detoxification Diet. Animal protein, meat, fish, poultry, eggs, and cheese, as well as cereal and nuts, with the exception of almonds, are acid forming.* These foods yield an acid ash after digestion. Too much of this acid ash becomes toxic to your cells and bodily fluids."

HIGHLY ALKALINE-FORMING FOODS	HIGHLY ACID-FORMING FOODS
Green leafy vegetables	Eggs
Soybeans	Smoked fish (herring)
Lima beans	Shell fish
Almonds	Fatty fish (sardines)
Carrots	Organ meats
Beets	Chicken
Potatoes	Beef
Buckwheat	Pork
Millet	Turkey

MILDLY ALKALINE-FORMING FOODS	MILDLY ACID-FORMING FOODS
Fresh fruit	Corn
Tomatoes	Cheese
Parsley	Legumes (except soybeans)
Green peas	Breads
String beans	Brown rice
Mushrooms Asparagus	Nuts (except almonds)

THE HI·LITE DIET TO THE RESCUE

"Mary Ellen, you need a highly alkaline nutritional program to correct your assimilation disorder. This is what detoxification is all
about. As your body becomes more alkaline, it, in turn, will have a
stabilizing influence on your mood changes. So be sure you are keeping your diet alkaline by eating plentiful supplies of alkaline fruit
salads and vegetable salads, raw vegetable juices, and fresh fruit
juices."

HIGHLY ALKALINE-FORMING JUICES
carrot-celery-spinach
carrot-celery-parsley
carrot-celery-beet
carrot-celery-cucumber

MILDLY ALKALINE
pineapple
grapefruit
orange
watermelon

Mary Ellen followed the Hi·Lite alkaline Cleansing Diet for one
week. She did very well. Once I was assured that the cleansing process was gaining momentum (she stayed on the diet), I switched her
into second gear. I told her she was ready for the Hi·Lite Detoxification Diet.

"Remember, in fact the Detoxification Diet is simply an expansion
of the fundamental Cleansing Diet. Its higher fiber content gives it
mechanical leverage to sweep out the acid poison from the bile ducts
to the intestines. You emphasize raw garden-fresh vegetable salads.
Add whole grains such a 7-grain sprouted breads, brown rice, millet,
and legumes such as soybeans, lima beans, and lentils to the cleansing program. Continue to leave out dairy products and flesh foods.
The Hi·Lite Maintenance Diet is then built upon the foundation of the
Cleansing Diet and the Detoxification Diet."

A typical day in the life of a Detoxification Diet is:

DETOXIFICATION DIET — A TYPICAL DAY

Breakfast:	(1)	Fresh, vibrant watermelon juice (6-8 oz.)
		15 minutes later:
	(2)	**MELON MEDLEY SALAD** with watermelon, cantaloupe, and honeydew topped with 1 Tbsp. almonds and ¼ cup **CRUNCHY GRANOLA.**
Mid-Morning:	(1)	Liver Detoxification Smoothie
Lunch:	(1)	Fresh carrot juice (8 oz.)
		15 minutes later:
	(2)	**COOL CUCUMBER SALAD** with romaine lettuce leaves, juicy ripe tomato slices, sprouts, crisp cucumber slices, and carrots, topped with **LEMON-GARLIC DRESSING** and 2 tsp. sesame seeds.
	(3)	1-2 slices 7-grain sprouted whole grain bread, pita bread, or corn tortillas. Eat with the salad or make into a **MELTZER B-L-T VEGETABLE SANDWICH** (bread, lettuce, tomato).

Mid-Afternoon:	(1)	Magic Detoxification Potion

Dinner:	(1)	Fresh carrot juice (8 oz.)
		15 minutes later:
	(2)	**THE MELTZER VEGETABLE SALAD SUPREME** with crisp romaine lettuce leaves, juicy ripe tomato slices, your favorite sprouts, red onion, cucumber, and sliced carrots, topped with **KELP·FROM·THE·SEA DRESSING.**
	(3)	**STEAMED GREEN VEGETABLE PLATTER** (asparagus, peas, string beans, etc.)
	(4)	**RICO VEGIE·RICE CASSEROLE*** with zucchini, broccoli, carrots, and brown rice.

---

*Refer to recipe section, page 95.

After one full week of cleansing and one week of detoxification, Mary Ellen started to feel a sense of emotional control. Her eyes were sparkling and her coloring was much improved. She went through emotional detoxification; that is, negative emotions that had been suppressed began to surface. Her warm, positive, loving nature reappeared. I then started her on the Hi·Lite Maintenance Diet.

Mary Ellen became so thoroughly involved with her new eating habits within two weeks of starting the program, she had cut down on her tranquilizers. After being on the Maintenance Diet for only four days, she got rid of all her pills. Her new body chemistry created the internal environment for feeling better. With the proper alkaline to acid ratio in her diet, the stiffness in her body, an early sign of rheumatism, disappeared.

With the help of her Detoxification Diet, Mary Ellen got in control of her emotional stress. While working through the process of detoxification, you become comfortably familiar with your inner thoughts and feelings. When Mary Ellen's body chemistry became more balanced, she started to experience her real personal belief systems.

Everybody has his own personal beliefs. You see, your beliefs are your strongest convictions. They are your personal feelings about what you accept as being true and real. You can only be committed to what you believe in. And your beliefs have an uncanny way of becoming a self-fulfilling prophecy.

When your nerves and your glands are not properly nourished, the toxemia of your mind and emotions causes you to fall victim to the dusky nightshade of the nutritional "twilight zone." With a mind that is not focused and emotions that are tied up with anxiety, it is very difficult to see that you have adopted negative beliefs about yourself.

Beneath the surface, Mary Ellen was deathly afraid of getting older. Her previous over-acid biochemical imbalance was causing her to feel out of it. When you are not in control of your thoughts and feelings, negative destructive belief systems can run your life. This is what happened to Mary Ellen. Both her parents had died in their fifties. When Mary Ellen started feeling bad and losing her pep, her negative beliefs about her impending senility and loneliness found little resistance in taking over her mind. With a renewed sense of mental clarity from her detoxification program, her positive, intuitive beliefs about herself began to thrive. She took command of her life by adding a daily jog and daily meditation to her health program before she had her breakfast. Her physical vitality and sense of mental well-being rejuvenated her self-confidence. The Detoxification Diet raised her consciousness. She became self-motivated. Her hi-enzyme, high alkaline nutritional program was a valued catalyst to her new-found positive mental and emotional hygiene.

Within a few months, Mary Ellen laid the ground work for a new permanent relationship. The one with herself. She realized that she loved her husband. She clarified her commitment and found out that loving him made her happy. She also determined that her needs for a close loving relationship could be met with her husband. With the channels of communication flowing, Mary Ellen straightened out her emotional life. And as long as she continues to pay respect to her Hi·Lite diet, she will stay well.

OPEN YOUR MIND

Detoxification promotes a healthy clear mind. In point of fact, detoxification diets work to purify and strengthen your mind. This enables you to be in intimate touch at a super-high level of communication with your true emotions. With an open mind and a loving heart, you can deal directly with your personal belief systems.

Experiencing positive beliefs about yourself is intuitive. When you get to know yourself, you can become very enthusiastic about being alive. You can know the importance of your own life and how natural it is to be happy, relaxed and healthy. As you get clear about what you need and want in your life, your beliefs will become self-evident. Taking the necessary action to stand up for what you believe in is more spontaneous and easier with the positive mental and emotional hygiene created by hi-enzyme, hi-alkaline Hi·Lite nutrition.

Changing personal belief systems from negative into positive ones can be accomplished through the powers of the emotional, spiritual, and mental detoxification process. This is aided and abetted by effective meditation and daily exercise. Clear-minded thinking and spiritual re-purification is necessary to facilitate and replace old thoughts about yourself with new, positive, constructive ones. The Hi·Lite Detoxification Program is conducive to getting to the core of your real personal belief systems and inspiring you to do something about them. This most special kind of internal communication is made possible when you take charge of your diet. This means becoming responsible for eating the best foods that will give you:

- *More spontaneous, loving feelings.*
- *Inner strength.*
- *A capacity to control negative emotions.*

The Hi·Lite Detox Diet is intended to create modest changes in your lifestyle. It relies on your self-motivation to place a higher premium on taking care of and nourishing yourself each day.

5: DETOXIFICATION DIET RECIPES

The Nutritional Detoxification Diet is built upon the backbone of the predominantly raw food cleansing diet. Detox calls for the addition of whole grain breads and cereals as well as selected cooked grains and legumes. The food preparation tips to help you stick to the detox plan will be found on the following pages.

FOOD GROUPS IA and IIA: Fresh Fruit and Raw Vegetable Juices

Pure living juices are a necessary requirement for the Detoxification Diet. Consult Cleansing Diet Recipes, pages 53-64, for details. Elixirs of rejuvenation are fundamental to the detox plan. Two pickups are recommended, one at 10:30 a.m. and the other at 3:30 p.m.

Liver Detoxification Smoothie

6-8 oz. fresh fruit juice
  or 1 cup fruit
1½ Tbsp. Brewers yeast

1 Tbsp. rice bran syrup
1 tsp. bee pollen

Mix above ingredients in a blender. Blend it well and drink it slowly.

Spirulina Surprise

8 oz. fresh raw carrot juice
1 tsp. spirulina

Mix above ingredients in blender. Drink slowly over five minutes.

FOOD GROUP I: Hi·Lite Fruit Salad Supremes

See Cleansing Diet, page 21. Emphasize the fruits in season. For example, melons in the summer, apples and pears in the fall, citrus in the winter, and berries in the spring.

FOOD GROUP II: Hi·Lite Crisp Leafy Green Chlorophyll Salads

The fundamentals of preparing fresh raw green vegetable salads remain the same. Tabouli, a bulgar-wheat based crisp refreshing salad, is an additional alternative:

Terrific Tabouli

(Fresh parsley is the secret to this mid-eastern luncheon treat)

1 cup bulgar wheat	1 stalk celery, chopped
½ green pepper, chopped	Juice from 1-3 lemons (to taste)
½ tomato, chopped	½ tsp. dill
½ cup fresh parsley, chopped	2 Tbsp. fresh mint leaves
3 cloves garlic, diced	3 green onions, chopped
½ cucumber, chopped	(or ½ red onion, chopped)

Bring 2 cups water to boil. Pour over bulgar, cover and let stand until all the water has been soaked up, 30 minutes. Strain off any additional water. Add balance of ingredients, stirring well. Refrigerate several hours or overnight to allow flavors to blend. Serve on a bed of lettuce, topped with alfalfa sprouts and lemon tahini dressing, or stuff inside pita bread.

FOOD GROUP III: Steamed Green Vegetable Combinations

The steamed vegetable combinations are the same as for the Cleansing Diet. See page 23.

FOOD GROUP IV: Selected Whole Grain Cereals

Try your hand at granola or a hearty bowl of oatmeal for breakfast.

Sharon's Crunchy Granola

(No oil is needed for a tasty, healthful granola.)

2 cups rolled oats	½ cup water
1 cup wheat flakes	1 tsp. cinnamon
⅓ cup honey	1 tsp. vanilla (optional)

Mix above ingredients together thoroughly and place on an ungreased cookie sheet. Bake at 250° for 1 hour, turning granola every 15 minutes. The granola will be soft when it comes out of the oven. Cool to let it crunch. Store in airtight container.

Cinnamon-Oat Cereal

(A warm, soothing cereal for those frosty fall mornings)

1 cup rolled oats
5-6 toasted almonds (5 or 6
    whole or can be ground in
    blender or nut grinder)

2 cups water
1 tsp. cinnamon
1 medium banana, sliced

Bring water to a rolling boil in covered pan. Stir in above ingredients, turn off heat, cover and let sit for 5-10 minutes, stirring occasionally. The banana imparts a sweetness, making the addition of honey unnecessary. You can also omit the banana and add honey to taste after the cereal is cooked.

Variation: Try adding 1 chopped unpeeled pippin apple in place of the banana.

Oatmeal

1¾ cups water
1 Tbsp. cinnamon
¼ cup raisins (optional)

2 Tbsp. soy grits
1⅓ cups steel cut rolled oats
Honey to taste

Bring water to boil. Add raisins and cinnamon while it heats. When boiling, add the soy grits and rolled oats. Lower heat and cook, uncovered, until the water is absorbed and the oats are just tender. (Mixture will become thick quite soon.) Add honey on top as desired.

FOOD GROUP V: Selected Whole Grain Breads

Baking bread has been a labor of love for men and women throughout the centuries. The art form of making your own breads has been captured in a number of New Age cookbooks. In general, first-rate markets or health food stores will carry all the whole grain bread selections of your Detox Diet.

FOOD GROUP VI: Selected Cooked Whole Grains

When cooking grains, use a pot with a tight-fitting lid. Bring water to boil in deep saucepan. Add grain slowly while stirring. Simmer recommended time. Do not stir during simmering stage. When cooked, all water should be absorbed by grain. Fluff lightly with two forks when cooked. Since pots and stoves vary, trial and error will tell you the correct cooking time. Therefore, times listed below are approximate. Be sure to drain in colander.

Cooking Times for Grains

Grain (1 cup dry)	Water	Cooking time
Barley, pearl	2½ cups	1 hour
Buckwheat groats, raw	3 cups	20-25 minutes
Cornmeal and corn grits	4 cups	30 minutes
Millet (saute in 1 Tbsp. oil for nutty flavor)	3 cups	30 minutes
Oats, whole	3 cups	1 hour
Oats, flaked or rolled	3 cups	30 minutes
Rice, sweet or short grain	2 cups	50 minutes
Rice, long grain	2 cups	40-50 minutes
Rye berries	2½ cups	1 hour
Rye flakes	2 cups	20 minutes
Triticale berries	2½ cups	20 minutes
Wheat berries	2½ cups	1 hour
Wheat, bulgar	2 cups	15-20 minutes
Wheat flakes	2 cups	20 minutes

For example, here is how to make your brown rice:

Brown Rice

Short, medium or long grain can be mixed together. Wild rice can be added and cooked with the other rices for added flavor. Add 1 bay leaf with your favorite herbs, such as dill and onion or add a vegetable boullion cube (or Tamari). As a rule of thumb, 1 part rice to 2 parts water. Cook 40-50 minutes. Cooked rice is 2½ times the quantity of uncooked rice.

Spanish Barley

1 cup barley
2½ cups water
¼ cup green pepper, chopped
¼ cup mushrooms, chopped

2-3 medium tomatoes, chopped and blended
Chopped onions, as desired
Cilantro, parsley, oregano are suggested seasonings

In a skillet, saute onion in oil. Add the barley, tomatoes, and stir gently while adding the water. Cover tightly and cook approximately 45-60 minutes. Add green pepper, mushrooms, and onion during last 10 minutes of cooking. Oregano and parsley or cilantro may be added for seasoning. Just place the vegetables on top of the barley to steam and fluff together when cooking is complete.

It is also possible to use your knowledge and prepare a variety of interesting vegetable-rice casseroles.

Rico Vegie-Rice Casserole

1 cup zucchini, sliced
1 cup broccoli, broken in flowerets
1 cup carrots, sliced
2 tomatoes, chopped

¼ cup onion, chopped
2 Tbsp. parsley, chopped
½ cup brown rice, raw
1 cup cold water

Steam lightly zucchini, broccoli, and carrots. Cook remaining ingredients with the brown rice for 40 minutes. Place alternate layers of steamed vegetables and rice mixture in casserole. Heat in 325° oven for 15 minutes. This is great for left-over rice — in that case, just saute tomatoes, onion, parsley, and celery in ½ Tbsp. olive oil and mix with left-over rice. Recipe can also use those left-over steamed vegetables.

GROUP VII: Selected Legumes

Knowing how to use tofu, lentils, and lima beans adds style and wholesome variety to your Detoxification Diet. Tofu is of the highest quality vegetable protein. Lima beans are alkaline and lentils are proteinacious.

Tofu soybean curd (also called soy cheese) is very versatile. Cube it and add it to soups, stews, and casseroles. It makes an excellent base for casseroles. Slice or cube it and add your favorite tomato sauce or gravy. Then bake and serve.

Here is how to scramble up your tofu:

Scrambled Tofu

3 Tbsp. safflower oil (unrefined)
1 onion, diced
2 cups tofu, cut into cubes
12-16 mushrooms, chopped

3 cloves garlic, crushed
1 Tbsp. fresh ginger, grated (optional)
1 cup mung bean or soybean sprouts (optional)
herbs of your choice (spike, tamari)

In a large skillet heat oil. Saute onion until golden brown. Add tofu. Cover and steam in own juices, stirring often. When lightly brown and tender, add mushrooms and seasonings. Cover and cook briefly. During the last few minutes of cooking, add sprouts (optional). Addition of water may be necessary.

Other vegetables may be included for vegetable chow mein. Serve over brown rice.

With a bit of tofu and brown rice, you can put together a delicious vegetarian chop suey:

Vegetarian Chop Suey

1 Tbsp. safflower oil
1 large onion, chopped
½ cup celery, chopped
1 cup mushrooms

1 cup mung bean sprouts
½ cup Chinese cabbage
Cubed tofu (½ lb.)

Saute onion and celery until almost soft. Add mushrooms, sprouts, and cabbage. Toss and saute for 3-5 minutes. Add tofu to heat. Serve over brown rice if desired. A small dash of tamari adds extra flavor. Also, 1 tsp. minced ginger may be added while you saute the vegetables. Broccoli, snow peas, or sesame seeds are other optional additions.

Another variation is to make tofu rice croquettes:

Sharon's Tofu-Rice Croquettes

1 cup brown rice, raw
1 lb. tofu
½ cup sesame seeds, ground
2-3 green onions, chopped

¼ cup parsley, chopped
1 clove garlic, pressed
Sesame oil, as needed to hold
    patties together
Tamari, to taste

Cook rice in 2 cups water (or use 2 cups cold left-over rice). Mash tofu with fork and mix balance of ingredients, adding oil if necessary. Form into patties and place on lightly oiled cookie sheet. Bake at 350° for 40 minutes. Turn over, sprinkle with paprika and broil until golden. Serve with yeast gravy.

For the sake of completion, just a few words on sauteeing your vegetables is in order.

Sauteed Vegetables

Use a wok, stainless steel or cast iron frypan with a lid. Place 1-2 Tbsp. cold-pressed safflower oil in the pan on medium-high heat. (When a treated cast iron pan is used, the oil can be omitted. Add water if sticking is a problem.) Add pressed garlic or chopped onion and stir. Add hardest vegetables first, stir, cover, turn heat to medium and cook 2-4 minutes. Add remaining vegetables, cover and cook just until tender. Practice makes perfect!

Tofu can also be used as a sandwich filling when blended with dill, caraway seed, chopped parsley, onion, and garlic. Try making a high-protein salad dressing by blending tofu with a small amount of oil and spices, including onion, garlic, parsley, tamari, and paprika. A cheese-cake-type mixture can be achieved by mixing honey with the tofu, some additional water, and vanilla flavoring.

Lima beans can be very tasty. Here's how:

Lani's Lima-Bean-Rice Soup

1 lb. dry lima beans, soaked
    4 hours
2 cups celery, with leaves, chopped
½ cup onion, chopped

2 cups tomato, chopped
2 Tbsp. olive oil
1 cup raw brown rice
Seasonings of choice

Cook lima beans with celery, onion, and tomato until almost tender. Keep water in your pan so beans are always covered. Add oil and rice when beans are almost tender. Continue cooking for one hour. Additional water may be added to achieve desired thickness.

Lima Bean — Mixed Vegetable Soup

1½ cups dried lima beans
1½ cups celery, chopped
1½ cups carrots, chopped
1½ cups onions, chopped
½ cup green pepper, finely
    chopped

1½ cups green beans, cut into
    2-inch pieces
2-3 tomatoes, chopped into small
    chunks
Water to cover ingredients by
    one inch.

Seasonings: Bay leaf, ½ tsp. black pepper, 2 Tbsp. apple cider vinegar, ½ tsp. kelp, basil.

Rinse and soak the beans overnight or for several hours in enough water to cover. Drain. Cook beans with bay leaf and enough water until tender. Add vegetables and cook until tender. Add tomato and seasonings at end. Before serving, remove ⅓ of liquid and blend in blender. Return to soup pot and reheat. Serve hot. Serves 6-8.

Lentil soup is a satisfying staple to a healthy Detoxification Diet.

Luscious Lentil Soup

1 cup dry lentils
1 bay leaf
1 red onion, chopped
1 stalk celery, chopped

1 carrot, sliced
2-3 tomatoes, blended with
    enough water to blend
8 mushrooms, sliced

Seasonings of choice: dill, ginger, cumin, cayenne, basil (¼ tsp. each), 2 cloves garlic.

Cook lentils and bay leaf in 2 cups water for 30 minutes. Add balance of ingredients and simmer until lentils are tender.

While you're learning about soups, how about Lani's Peanut Soup:

Lani's Peanut Soup

4 Tbsp. peanut butter,
    roasted smooth
4 Tbsp. onions, chopped
2 Tbsp. celery, chopped

½ tsp. raw ginger
1 cup water
Tamari to taste
Chives for garnish on top

Blend peanut butter with ginger, water, and tamari. Heat but do not allow to boil. Add onion and celery and simmer, covered, 20 minutes.

FOOD GROUP VIII: Salad Dressings

All your choice dressings on the Cleansing Diet are acceptable. Here are two more for variety:

Lemon-Tahini Dressing

1 cup lemon juice (may be
    substituted in part with cider
    vinegar)
1¾ cup combined olive and
    safflower oil
1 large clove garlic, crushed
pinch black pepper

1 tsp. basil
½ tsp. oregano
½ tsp. marjoram
pinch of celery seed
Fresh parsley, finely chopped
Juice from 1 orange
½ cup tahini

Combine all ingredients and chill to blend flavors.

Gourmet Tarragon Dressing

¼ cup vegetable oil
2-3 Tbsp. apple cider vinegar
½ tsp. tamari sauce

1 clove garlic, pressed
2 Tbsp. tarragon
¼ cup water

Mix in blender. Chill one hour.

6: THE MAINTENANCE DIET

Building up your body Chemistry

The Hi·Lite Nutritional Maintenance Diet builds up your body. It keeps you in possession of your most vital faculties. It also keeps you sharp, agile, and bright. The Nutritional Maintenance Diet is for everyone, including the infant, the elderly, the teenager, and the mature adult. It works for the businessman, the housewife, the pregnant mother, the laborer, the professional in the city, and the cowboy in the country.

The Maintenance Diet frames the right structure into place for longevity and illness-free living. The maintenance plan essentially establishes you as a healthy, vital human being capable of reaching out to others. The abundance of the Hi·Lite Nutritional Maintenance Diet is seen in your top-flight energy level.

The essence of the Maintenance Diet lies in its balance. The diet provides all the essential nutrients for optimal human nourishment. The purpose of the diet is to safely organize your body chemistry. The Maintenance Diet deliberately assembles high-quality micronutrients into the proper food combinations for optimal organic cellular function.

There is an intelligent rhyme and reason to the Maintenance Diet. The diet has the ability to cleanse and detoxify your system while supporting your growth and development at the same time. The anatomy of the Hi·Lite maintenance plan takes into consideration the natural elements of nutritional mending. The Maintenance Diet has:

- *a cleansing foundation*
- *a detoxification background*
- *high-quality nutritive fiber for elimination of waste and garbage*
- *restorative, transforming, nourishing hi-enzyme life-giving principles*
- *purification powers*
- *a regular juice fasting program*

Therefore, you can say that the Maintenance Diet is a cleansing diet, a detoxification diet, an elimination diet, a replacement diet, and a restorative diet all rolled into one. That is why it is so effective in keeping you well.

The balancing effect of the diet is very conducive to the integration of your whole being, at all levels. The desire of the Maintenance Diet is to sustain the unification of mind, body, and spirit that stands for outstanding health.

IMPROVE YOUR SEX LIFE

The Maintenance Diet will invariably improve your sex life. With a greater sense of nutritional balance, you will feel and be more potent. Women who for years have been trying to get pregnant find themselves pregnant and bearing a child while following this maintenance plan. Men who have complained of sexual ineptness find themselves attractive and virile. The balancing effect the Maintenance Diet has on your bodily hormones is physiologically and mentally responsible for your more active sex drive and stronger sex life.

To be solid, steady and firm is the theme of the nutritional maintenance plan. The program gives you the grip to call your own shots. The power of the nutritional maintenance plan provides you with the control to keep the ball rolling in your corner of the world. Before starting the diet consult the Physiology and Hi·lights of Nutritional Maintenance.

PHYSIOLOGY OF THE 7-DAY
HI·LITE MAINTENANCE PROGRAM

HI·LITE NUTRITIONAL MAINTENANCE: BUILD IT UP

DAY 15	RE·VIVE IT	**TRANS·FUSE IT**
DAY 16	REL·BIRTH IT	**TRANS·PLANT IT**
DAY 17	RE·CONSTRUCT IT	**RE·STOCK IT**
DAY 18	REPLACE IT	**RE·STORE IT**
DAY 19	RE·CREATE IT	**RE·GENERATE IT**
DAY 20	REFINE·IT	**RE·HABILITATE IT**
DAY 21	RE·JUVENATE IT	**MEND IT**

DAY 15: REVIVE IT

When your diet maintains its course, it gets you where you want to go. The weekly schedule of the Hi·Lite Maintenance Plan begins with a full day of juice fasting. The hi-enzyme Hi·Lite energy of this quality liquid-only diet pours new vibrant energy into your circulation, lymph and bodily fluids. Juicing·it·up transfuses fresh new life into your veins.

DAY 16: RE·BIRTH IT

The balanced chemistry of the Maintenance Diet lays down the seeds to harvest fitness and vitality. The diet plants the right food nutrients into the soil of your body chemistry. The nourishment of the diet stimulates your whole being to take a turn for the better. The transport of superior nutrition into your cells is conducive to the flowering and the lush blossoming of your system. In effect, this trans·plants you into a heightened sensitivity and a new level of well-being. It also establishes an internally gratifying way of life.

DAY 17: RE·CONSTRUCT IT

The rhythmic hi-enzyme Maintenance Diet is designed to re·stock your body's warehouse of vitamins, minerals, essential amino acids, and unsaturated fatty acids. This is accomplished by eating a variety of fresh, living, wholesome foods. The diet includes a heavier dose of whole grains, legumes, and complete protein to firmly reconstitute nuclei and cell membranes. The maintenance plan efficiently reconstructs enzymes, hormones, and neurochemical transmitters. This rebuilds your metabolic machinery at the same time you are cleaning out the hardware.

DAY 18: REPLACE IT

In effect, the consistency and continuity of the Hi·Lite maintenance plan restores harmony in your body chemistry. It improves your condition. It restores integrity to the altar of your healing. It favorably reinstates peak efficiency to the throne of your well-being. It puts you back into shape and brings you back to consciousness.

DAY 19: RE·CREATE IT

In short order, the Maintenance Diet biochemically regenerates living cells and tissues into a new reality. Regeneration is, in fact, a new beginning. In this way the maintenance plan recreates a spiritual and physiological rebirth. In a way it completely reforms your whole body. It re-establishes an inner strength that generates more and more power. This is the basis for the ongoing, seemingly effortless and yet endless energy level of the maintenance plan.

DAY 20: RE·FINE IT

The Hi·Lite Maintenance Diet is said to be the dietary passageway to total re·habilitation. It therefore serves not only for those who want to stay well, but also for those who are on the road to recovery. Rehabilitation takes into consideration how to patch up burned out nerves, glands, and hormones that have suffered emotional stress, mental strain, and spiritual *darkness.*

DAY 21: RE·JUVENATE IT

The upshot of this nutritional transformation is manifested in a natural physiological mending. In effect, the Maintenance Diet reinstates vitality to your nerves, vim to your heart, and vigor to your soul. It gives you the get-up-and-go that you've always wanted. In reality, the Maintenance Diet mends your ways. Your health improves for the better. Damaged parts become fit for use. Nutritional mending makes you whole. Wear and tear is turned into sound privileged function. Applying the Maintenance Diet on a daily basis totally corrects your health.

The Maintenance Diet upholds the principles of a balanced maintenance regime by adhering to the natural food distribution within the four major food groups:

- 50% Simple Natural Carbohydrates
- 15-20% Whole Complex Carbohydrates
- 15-20% High Quality Complete Protein
- 15-20% Natural Fats

The Maintenance Diet, therefore is a high natural carbohydrate, high fiber, low fat, moderate protein diet. This is the right amount of protein. The caloric value ranges anywhere from 1800 to 2500+ calories, depending upon your lifestyle and habits.

Maintenance has Enough Protein

Keep in mind that the Maintenance Diet has substantial amounts of complete protein. It is carefully constructed so that no less than 70% be of vegetable protein origin and no greater than 30% be animal protein. The addition of animal protein, as well as animal fat, is one of the distinguishing features of the Maintenance Diet. This diet provides flexible quantities of high-quality complete protein, ranging anywhere from 30 to 60 gms. or more to match your needs. Although the cleansing and detoxifying Hi·Lite dietary programs are strictly vegetarian, the Maintenance Diet offers you the option to go vegetarian or not. The lacto-vegetarian maintenance diet is the recommended form of the Hi·Lite maintenance program. The nonvegetarian alternative will be explained later in the Guidelines of the Maintenance Diet.

You can be sure you are getting enough protein when you feel good, are energetic, and can sustain a happy, active sex life. Your body needs just the right amount of protein, not too much and not too little. That is what balance is all about.

THE BIOCHEMICAL ESSENCE OF THE HI·LITE HI-ENZYME MAINTE-NANCE DIET IS TO COMBINE RAW LIVING FOOD WITH COMPLETE PROTEIN AT EACH AND EVERY MEAL.

Vegetarians can get enough high-quality protein by following the complete protein dietary exchanges outlined in the maintenance program. How will you live without meat? Very well and very happily. In general, most adults require 50 gms. of protein to sufficiently maintain daily protein needs built into their American lifestyle. This does not apply to children and teenagers under the age of 18 years.

NUTRITIONAL SUPPLEMENTS FOR MAINTENANCE

ALL PURPOSE COMPREHENSIVE VITAMIN-CHELATED

MINERAL SUPPLEMENT: (AS DIRECTED FOR DAILY CONSUMPTION)

HI-POTENCY B COMPLEX	1 with breakfast (or lunch) and 1 with dinner
VITAMIN C (ROSE HIPS WITH BIOFLAVINOIDS)	500 mg 2 x day
VITAMIN E (mixed tocopherols)	400 I.U. 15 minutes before breakfast and 15 minutes before dinner
BREWERS YEAST	1½ Tbsp 2 x day

Most certainly, there are ample opportunities to get enough vitamin B-12 on the Maintenance Diet. With your consumption of dairy products, aged cheese, sunflower seeds, kelp, bananas, peanut butter, bee pollen, tempeh or spirulina, you can be certain to get enough B-12. Also, brewers yeast is often fortified with B-12, and most all-purpose nutritional supplement will carry a daily minimum of 100 mcg. of B-12. Important trace minerals such as chromium, selenium and manganese will be available with the raw foods, complete protein, and above nutritional supplements.

One word about cheating while on this diet. As we were taught in grade school, the only person you really cheat when you are cheating is yourself. When you are on the Cleansing and Detoxification Diets, it is important for you to go through all the fundamental steps of staying on this program. To get the main benefits of the diet, the closer you follow it, the more benefits you will receive. And it is not a direct linear phenomenon. In other words, by following the Cleansing or Detoxification or Maintenance Diet 50% you don't necessarily get 50% results. By following the diet 60% you don't necessarily get 60% results. The main benefit comes from the continuity and consistency of following the diet at least 85% of the way. Otherwise, you won't really ever know what your potential is to experience the benefits of this dietary program. As you get in touch with your own dietary and emotional needs, you become more of an expert in determining what your optimal diet is.

Keep cool. Be discrete. Stay relaxed and centered. Then you will know what to do.

When You Travel Or Go Out

When you are traveling, keep an open mind. With seeing eyes, you can stay as close to nature as is possible. Seek out the best natural food restaurants. Ask around, and look up specialized dining-out directories to find out the best places to eat. When you go out to eat, especially when you are with friends, enjoy yourself.

Have fun. And be sure to place the highest priority on loving, sharing, and communication. The food you are eating is not the main reason why you are with your friends. When people ask you why you are "dieting" you can simply respond that you feel better eating what appeals to you. With a smile on your face and Light in your eyes, tell them it's really quite a lot of fun for you to eat what you are eating. Just be mellow and calm about it.

With some creativity, persistence, and enthusiasm, you can usually find some high quality restaurants. It all boils down to your values and what it is that you are looking for. Be clear about what it is in nutrition that turns you on. Absolutely draw the lines on what you will and will not eat. And then within the boundaries of what you allow yourself to eat, enjoy.

Individuals in good health can maintain **great** health on the Hi·Lite Maintenance Diet. Remember, there are four nutritional wheels to the winged chariot of the Hi·Lite Del Mar Diet. In conjunction with the Fasting Regime, the Cleansing Diet, and the Detoxification Diet, the Maintenance Diet rounds out the field. Combined with a regular exercise routine, a balanced lifestyle, and a daily meditation program, the reader who wants to achieve optimal, vibrant wellness is on his way. Then simply completely relax emotionally to be at one with yourself. Turn to your Nutritional Hi·Lights for the details. The Hi·Lights will help you stick to the diet.

Seasonal Fresh Fruit and Fruit Juices	yes	All fresh fruits in season. **FRESH FRUIT SALAD SUPREME** at breakfast. Fruit salad option available for lightweight lunch. Emphasis on apples, canteloupe, oranges, bananas, pineapples, grapefruit, peaches. Dried fruits in moderation for social occasions.
Fresh Vegetables and Raw Vegetable Juices	yes	All fresh vegetables with emphasis on mushrooms, fresh peas, celery, carrots, avocado, cauliflower, romaine lettuce, sprouts, spinach, tomatoes, red onions, cucumber. Steamed broccoli, zucchini, string bean and eggplant are of significance.
Sprouts	yes	Emphasize alfalfa and bean sprouts with your raw salads.
Nuts	yes	Almonds, walnuts, and cashews in moderation. Pecans, brazil nuts, and macadamia nuts for special occasions. Absolutely no salt. Follow precautions on Cleansing Diet.
Nut Butter	yes	Peanut butter, cashew butter, almond butter, sesame-tahini butter, unsalted and unhydrogenated.
Seeds	yes	Sunflower, sesame, or pumpkin seeds as a garnish to your vegetable salad.
Natural Starchy Carbohydrates	yes	One night a week, at least, recommended on Maintenance Diet.
Whole grains	yes	Whole-grain cereals optional at breakfast. Whole-grain breads optional at lunch. Cooked whole grain optional at dinner. Eat whole grains at least 2 meals per day.
Legumes	yes	Tofu, soyburgers, beans, peas, and lentils are staples.
Total Dairy Intake		Up to once a day, no more than 2-3 times a week.
Daily Products: Milk	yes	Low-fat raw milk, low-fat buttermilk, up to once a day, no more than 2-3 times a week.
Cheese	yes	Avoid all pasteurized, processed, colored hard cheeses. Rennetless or raw cheese is the preferred high-fat cheese. Acceptable no more than 2-3 times a week.
Low-fat dairy	yes	Skim milk cheese, low-fat cottage cheese up to once a day, no more than 2-3 times a week.
Non-fat yogurt	yes	Up to once a day, no more than 2-3 times a week.
Flesh Foods: Meat **Fish or Chicken**	not recommended	The non-vegetarian alternative to the Meltzer Maintenance Diet is organic white meat of turkey without skin, organic white meat of chicken without skin, broiled or baked fish (except shellfish), or fertile eggs. Not more than once a day and up to 2-3 times a week.
Beverages	yes	Herbal teas of choice. Fresh fruit juices and one fresh carrot juice (8 oz.) per day.
Seasonings	yes	Cleansing herbs and the basic 7 herbs.
Supplements	yes	Emphasis on brewers yeast, B-complex vitamins, all-purpose comprehensive vitamin-and chelated mineral supplement, vitamin E, vitamin C.

HI· LIGHTS OF NUTRITIONAL MAINTENANCE — II.

The Blueprint For The Maintenance Diet

Morning:
Good Morning!
20 minutes of aerobics, deep breathing, and water initiation, followed by

Cosmic Interlude
15-20 minutes of yoga and meditation

THE MAINTENANCE BREAKFAST (7:00-8:00 a.m.)
(1) Fresh Fruit juice in season. (6 oz.)
     15 minutes followed by:
(2) **HI·LITE FRUIT SALAD SUPREME**
(3) COMPLETE PROTEIN FRUIT EXCHANGE*
(4) Alfalfa sprouts — optional (as many as you want)

Mid-Afternoon:
Sunshine, recharge your body, re-purify your mind, followed by:

Cosmic Interlude
THE MAINTENANCE LUNCHEON (12:30-2:00 p.m.) (Lunch is optional)

LIGHTWEIGHT	WELTERWEIGHT	HEAVYWEIGHT
Option 1: (1) **HI·LITE FRUIT SALAD SUPREME** (2) LIGHTWEIGHT FRUIT COMPLETE PROTEIN EXCHANGE	(1) **HI·LITE LEAFY-GREEN CHLOROPHYLL SALAD** (2) HERBAL SALAD DRESSING (3) WELTERWEIGHT LUNCHEON COMPLETE PROTEIN EXCHANGE	(1) **HI·LITE LEAFY-GREEN CHLOROPHYLL SALAD** (2) HERBAL SALAD DRESSING (3) HEAVYWEIGHT LUNCHEON COMPLETE PROTEIN EXCHANGE
Option 2: (1) **HI·LITE LEAFY-GREEN CHLOROPHYLL SALAD** (2) HERBAL SALAD DRESSING (3) LIGHTWEIGHT VEGETABLE COMPLETE PROTEIN EXCHANGE		

Evening:
15 minutes yoga and meditation

Cosmic Interlude
THE MAINTENANCE DINNER (5:00-7:00 p.m.)
(1) Fresh raw carrot juice, carrot-celery juice, or carrot-celery-beet juice
     15 minutes later
(2) **HI·LITE LEAFY-GREEN CHLOROPHYLL SALAD**, with your choice of:
(3) HERBAL SALAD DRESSING
     plus **one:**
(4) COMPLETE PROTEIN DINNER EXCHANGE

* COMPLETE PROTEIN EXCHANGES are **COMBINATIONS** of two or more foods that provide all the essential amino acids necessary to create a complete protein. There is a wide variety of acceptable Complete Protein Exchanges on the Maintenance Diet. Please refer to GROUP 7, pages 108-110.

The Maintenance Diet provides you with substantial amounts of essential protein that you need to stay in good health. When the right food ingredients of the Maintenance Diet are combined together appropriately with respect for the laws of food combining, nine fundamental food groups exist.

HI·LIGHTS OF NUTRITIONAL MAINTENANCE — III.

Food Groupings For The Maintenance Diet

GROUP 1:   **HI·LITE FRESH FRUIT SALAD SUPREMES**
Fall, Winter, Spring, and Summer are your four options. All the selections from the Cleansing Diet are acceptable.

GROUP 1a: **FRESH FRUIT JUICES:**
The fruit juice choices are the same as for the Cleansing and Detoxification Diets.

GROUP 2:   **HI·LITE LEAFY-GREEN CHLOROPHYLL SALADS**
All selections from the Cleansing Diet and the Detoxification Diet are acceptable.

GROUP 2a: **FRESH RAW VEGETABLE JUICES**
The choices are the same as for the Cleansing and Detoxification Diets. Carrot-celery-parsley or fresh tomato juice are also acceptable.

GROUP 3:   **COMPLETE PROTEIN FRUIT EXCHANGES**

A HI·LITE FRUIT SALAD SUPREME with any **one** of the following will make breakfast into a complete protein meal
   (1) 1 oz. almonds with 2 oz. granola
   (2) 1-2 Tbsp. nut butter with 2 oz. granola
   (3) 1-2 slices sprouted 7-grain bread with 1-2 Tbsp. nut butter
   (4) 1 oz. almonds with half a bowl 7-grain cereal, oatmeal, millet, bran, cream-of-rye or cream-of-wheat cereal
   (5) 1-3 oz. mixed nuts

GROUP 4:   **LIGHTWEIGHT LUNCHEON COMPLETE PROTEIN EXCHANGES**

GROUP 4a: **LIGHTWEIGHT FRUIT LUNCHEON COMPLETE PROTEIN EXCHANGE**

A HI·LITE FRUIT SALAD SUPREME with any **one** of the following will make a complete protein:
   (1) ½ cup low-fat cottage cheese
   (2) ½ cup non-fat yogurt
   (3) 1-3 oz. nuts and seeds
   (4) **MELTZER LIGHTWEIGHT FRUIT SMOOTHIE** (Take any Fruit Salad Supreme using appropriate seasonal fruits and blend together with 1-2 Tbsp. brewers yeast and 1 tsp. bee pollen.)

GROUP 4b: **LIGHTWEIGHT VEGETABLE LUNCHEON COMPLETE PROTEIN EXCHANGE**

A HI·LITE LEAFY-GREEN CHLOROPHYLL SALAD plus any **one** of the following will make a complete protein:
   (1) Raw carrots, peas, mushrooms, and 2 tsp. sunflower seeds added to salad.
   (2) Raw carrots, peas, cauliflower, and 2 tsp. sunflower seeds added to salad.
   (3) ½ cup steamed carrots, ½ cup steamed peas, 8 medium mushrooms and 2 tsp. sunflower seeds added to salad.
   (4) 1 cup steamed green vegetables of the season with 2 tsp. sunflower seeds added to raw sprouted salad.

GROUP 5: **WELTERWEIGHT LUNCHEON COMPLETE PROTEIN EXCHANGES**

A **HI·LITE LEAFY·GREEN CHLOROPHYLL SALAD** plus any **one** of the following will make a complete protein:

(1) **TERRIFIC TABOULI** with 2 tsp. sunflower seeds added to raw salad.
(2) **TOFU SALAD** with tofu, celery, onions, and tomato.
(3) **LANI'S LIMA BEAN RICE SOUP** with 2 tsp. sunflower seeds in salad.
(4) **BEAN VEGETABLE SOUP** with 2 tsp. sunflower seeds in salad.
(5) **SPICY SPLIT PEA SOUP** with 2 tsp. sunflower seeds in salad.
(6) **MIGHTY MUSHROOM AND CARROT·ONION SOUP** with sunflower or sesame seeds in salad.
(7) **LUSCIOUS LENTIL SOUP** with 2 tsp. sunflower seeds in salad.
(8) **PICES POTATO SALAD** (eggless) with 2 tsp. sunflower seeds.
(9) **OLD WORLD POTATO·LEEK SOUP** with cottage cheese (½ cup) with the salad.
(10) **WHOLLY GUACAMOLE** (avocado salad).
(11) **VEGETARIAN TACO** (fresh raw or steamed vegetables inside a warm corn tortilla).
(12) **AVOCADO SANDWICH** on 2 slices of sprouted 7-grain bread.
(13) **THE PITA STUFF** (avocado, tomato, sprouts, and onions inside whole wheat pita bread).
(14) **LAKE TACO,** wholly guacamole taco on corn tortilla or whole wheat chapati (guacamole taco without cheese).

GROUP 6: **HEAVYWEIGHT LUNCHEON COMPLETE PROTEIN EXCHANGES**

A **HI·LITE LEAFY·GREEN CHLOROPHYLL SALAD** plus any **one** of the following will make a complete protein:

(1) **AVOCADO SANDWICH** on 2 slices of sprouted 7-grain bread, and mixed vegetable soup.
(2) **AVOCADO SANDWICH** with choice of vegetable, bean, or pea soup.
(3) **THE PITA STUFF** (avocado, tomato, sprouts, and onions inside whole wheat pita bread), and mixed vegetable soup.
(4) **LUSCIOUS LENTIL SOUP** with 1-2 slices sprouted 7-grain bread.
(5) **MID·EASTERN GARBANZO SPREAD** (Hommus) with whole wheat pita bread.
(6) **TERRIFIC TABOULI** stuffed inside whole wheat pita bread.
(7) **WHOLLY GUACAMOLE** with vegetable bean soup.
(8) **LAKE TACO,** a guacamole taco on corn tortilla or whole wheat chapati without cheese, and mixed vegetable soup.
(9) **RAMONA'S QUESADILLA,** a corn tortilla with cheese, with or without mixed vegetable soup.
(10) **FEELING GREAT FILAFEL,** a garbanzo bean patty inside whole wheat pita bread.
(11) **LANI'S LIMA BEAN·RICE SOUP** with 1-2 slices sprouted 7-grain or whole wheat pita bread.
(12) **VEGE·BURGER:** Mushroom, soy, lentil, garbanzo, or tofu burger without bread with vegetable bean soup.
(13) **VEGE·BURGER** with whole wheat bun.
(14) **SPICY SPLIT PEA SOUP** with 1-2 slices sprouted 7-grain or whole wheat pita bread.
(15) **BEAN VEGETABLE SOUP** with 1-2 slices sprouted 7-grain or whole wheat pita bread.
(16) **MIGHTY MUSHROOM·CARROT·ONION SOUP** with 1-2 slices sprouted 7-grain or whole wheat pita bread.

GROUP 7: **COMPLETE DINNER PROTEIN EXCHANGES**

A **FRESH SPROUTED·GARDEN SALAD** with any one of the following will make a complete protein:

The 21·Day Del Mar Diet

GROUP 7a: COMPLETE CLEANSING EXCHANGES

    (1) 2-3 steamed vegetables in a mixed green vegetable platter, 1 baked potato, 2 tsp. sunflower seeds added to raw vegetable salad.

    (2) 2 steamed vegetables with corn on the cob; 2 tsp. sunflower seeds added to raw vegetable salad.

    (3) 2-3 steamed vegetables or mixed vegetable soup with baked yam or squash; 2 tsp. sunflower seeds added to salad.

GROUP 7b: COMPLETE TOFU EXCHANGES

    (1) 4 oz. scrambled tofu, 4 medium mushrooms, sauteed.

    (2) 4 oz. scrambled tofu, ½ cup wild rice, brown rice, or wild brown rice mixture.

    (3) **Vegetarian chop suey** with 4 oz. scrambled tofu, ½ cup wild or brown rice, plus mung bean sprouts, chinese cabbage, mushrooms, celery, onions.

    (4) Tofu-vegetable-mushroom-tice casserole with 4 oz. tofu, green vegetables, mushrooms, and brown rice.

    (5) **Rico-Vegie Rice Casserole** with 4 oz. tofu, and sauteed mushrooms.

    (6) 2 oz. tofu with mixed vegetable-rice soup.

    (7) Potato salad (eggless) with 2-3 oz. scrambled tofu and steamed vegetables.

    (8) **Tofu-Burger.**

GROUP 7c: COMPLETE SOYBEAN EXCHANGES

    (1) **Soybean brown rice vegetable casserole:** ½ cup cooked soybeans, ½ cup cooked brown rice or wild rice.

    (2) **Soyburger or Sesame-Soyburger.**

    (3) **Soyburger on whole grain bun.**

    (4) **Soy-cheeseburger.**

    (5) **Soy-cheeseburger with whole grain bun.**

    (6) ½ cup soy grits with ½ cup cooked brown rice.

    (7) 1 Soyburger made into soyballs with whole grain noodle vegetarian spaghetti.

GROUP 7d: COMPLETE BEAN EXCHANGES

    (1) **Organic tostada:** corn tortilla, ½ cup cooked beans (kidney and pinto), onions, tomato, sprouts.

    (2) **Filafel:** ¼ cup garbanzo beans made into a patty with mushrooms, onions, green bell pepper, and sesame seeds with or without pita bread.

    (3) **Hommus Lebanese Dip:** ½ cup cooked garbanzo bean spread, 1-2 slices whole wheat pita bread.

    (4) Beans (mung beans, aduki beans, lima beans, kidney beans, pinto beans) with brown or wild rice, ½ cup each.

GROUP 7e: COMPLETE SOUP AND GRAIN EXCHANGES

    (1) Lima bean vegetable soup, with 1-2 slices whole grain bread.

    (2) Lima bean vegetable soup, with brown rice.

    (3) Split pea soup, with ½ cup brown or wild rice.

    (4) Split pea soup, 1 bowl, with 1-2 slices whole grain or whole wheat pita bread.

    (5) Minestrone-bean-vegetable soup, with ½ cup brown rice.

    (6) Minestrone-bean-vegetable soup, with 1-2 slices whole grain bread.

    (7) Whole grain spaghetti noodles with tomato sauce and creamy mushroom soup.

    (8) Whole grain spaghetti noodles with natural tomato sauce, mixed with scrambled tofu and cream of beet soup (optional).

GROUP 7f: COMPLETE LENTIL EXCHANGES
    (1) Lentil-mixed vegetable soup with raw or sauteed mushrooms.
    (2) Lentil-mushroom-vegetable casserole with sesame or sunflower seeds in the salad.
    (3) Lentil-sesame or lentil-cashew nut roast.
    (4) Lentil soup with 1-2 slices whole grain or whole wheat pita bread.
    (5) Lentil soup with ½ cup brown rice or millet.
    (6) Lentil burger on whole wheat bun.

GROUP 7g: COMPLETE PEA EXCHANGES
    (1) Steamed carrots, steamed peas, 1 baked potato with 2 tsp. sesame seeds added to raw vegetable salad.
    (2) Vegetable casserole with steamed peas, mushrooms, and steamed greens with ½ cup brown rice, and sesame seeds (2 tsp.) added to raw salad.
    (3) Steamed peas, ½ cup, marinated mixed-bean salad, ¼ cup, 2 tsp. sesame seeds added to raw vegetable bean salad.

GROUP 7h: COMPLETE VEGETABLE-GRAIN CASSEROLES
    (1) Stuffed Bell Peppers with brown rice or millet.
    (2) **Indian Vegetable Curry** with brown rice or millet.
    (3) Balinese Tempeh in mushroom sauce.

GROUP 7i: VEGETABLE-CHEESE CASSEROLES
    (1) Eggplant-rice-cheese casserole.
    (2) **Eggplant Parmesan.**
    (3) Zucchini-rice-cheese casserole.
    (4) Green vegetable-rice-cheese casserole.
    (5) Carol's eggplant lasagna or artichoke lasagna.
    (6) **Vegetarian Pita Pizza.**

GROUP 7j: LOW-FAT DAIRY EXCHANGES
(Low-fat yogurt, farmer's cheese, ricotta cheese, skim milk or mozzarella cheese, buttermilk, hoop cheese, low-fat cottage cheese)
    (1) Steamed green vegetables, 1 baked potato and one serving from above.
    (2) Mixed vegetable minestrone bean soup with one low-fat dairy exchange.
    (3) Eggplant Parmesan with ricotta cheese.
    (4) **Ratatouille** with low-fat dairy products.
    (5) **Vegetarian pizza** with skim milk, farmer's or mozzarella cheese.

GROUP 7k: DAIRY EXCHANGES
(Raw or rennetless cheddar, colby, jack cheese)
    (1) **Cheese enchiladas** with ½ cup brown rice.
    (2) Quesadillas (corn tortillas with melted cheese) with vegetable soup.
    (3) Quesadilla with beans.
    (4) **Spinach Enchiladas**

GROUP 8: MAINTENANCE SALAD DRESSINGS
Select any HERBAL SALAD DRESSING from the Cleansing and Detoxification Diets. Additional salad dressing on the Maintenance Diet include:
    (1) **HERBAL YOGURT DRESSING**
    (2) **COWBOY RANCH DRESSING**
    (3) The Original "I" STREET YEAST GRAVY.
    (4) Salsa Picante

GROUP 9: MAINTENANCE DIET DESSERTS
    (1) **Crispy Apple Treat**
    (2) **Tasty Toasted Almond Fruit Pie Crust**
    (3) **Crusty Wheat Germ Fruit Pie**

HI· LIGHTS OF NUTRITIONAL MAINTENANCE — IV.

Golden Rules For The Maintenance Diet

The Maintenance Diet is simple to follow. The rules are:

RULE 1:
- EAT AT LEAST TWO MEALS A DAY: BREAKFAST AND LUNCH, OR BREAKFAST AND DINNER.

RULE 2:
- BREAKFAST BETWEEN 7:00 to 8:00 a.m. FOR 30 MINUTES.
- Select 6 oz. of **Fresh Fruit Juice** in season from **Group 1a**.
  15 minutes later:
- Choose 1 **FRUIT SALAD SUPREME** from **Group 1** in accordance with the appropriate season.
- Add 1 **COMPLETE PROTEIN FRUIT EXCHANGE** from **Group 3**.

RULE 3:
- LUNCH BETWEEN 12:30 and 2:00 p.m. IS OPTIONAL ON THE MAINTENANCE DIET.

  For those who have exerted themselves physically as well as mentally, a heavyweight luncheon is sometimes needed. For those who have exerted themselves mentally and not physically, at the best, a welterweight lunch is needed. For those that have neither exerted themselves physically or mentally, a lightweight luncheon will suffice. For those who have been rather inactive, don't feel compelled to eat lunch.

  (a) **For Lightweight Luncheon:**
  - Select 1 **FRUIT SALAD SUPREME** from **Group 1**.
  - Add 1 **LIGHTWEIGHT FRUIT LUNCHEON COMPLETE PROTEIN EXCHANGE** from **Group 4a**.
                      OR
  - Select 1 **LEAFY-GREEN CHLOROPHYLL SALAD** from **Group 2**.
  - Choose 1 **HERBAL SALAD DRESSING** from **GROUP 8**.
  - Add 1 **LIGHTWEIGHT VEGETABLE LUNCHEON COMPLETE PROTEIN EXCHANGE** from **Group 4b**.

  (b) **For Welterweight Luncheon:**
  - Select 1 **LEAFY-GREEN CHLOROPHYLL SALAD** from **Group 2**.
  - Choose 1 **HERBAL SALAD DRESSING** from **Group 8**.
  - Add 1 **WELTERWEIGHT LUNCHEON COMPLETE PROTEIN EXCHANGE** from **Group 5**.

  (c) **For Heavyweight Luncheon:**
  - Select 1 **LEAFY-GREEN CHLOROPHYLL SALAD** from **Group 2**.
  - Choose 1 **HERBAL SALAD DRESSING** from **Group 8**.
  - Add 1 **HEAVYWEIGHT LUNCHEON COMPLETE PROTEIN EXCHANGE** from **Group 6**.

RULE 4:
- DINE BETWEEN 5:00 and 7:00 p.m. ALLOW AT LEAST 30 MINUTES AND UP TO 90 MINUTES FOR A PLEASANT, ENJOYABLE DINNER.
- Drink 8 oz. **Fresh Vegetable Juice** from **Group 2b**.
- Choose 1 **LEAFY-GREEN CHLOROPHYLL SALAD** from **Group 2**.
- Add 1 **HERBAL SALAD DRESSING** from **Group 8**.
- Select 1 **COMPLETE DINNER PROTEIN COMBINATION** from **Group 7**:

A. CLEANSING PROTEINS	G. PEA PROTEINS
B. TOFU PROTEIN	H. VEGETABLE-GRAIN
C. SOYBEAN PROTEIN	PROTEINS
D. BEAN PROTEIN	I. VEGETABLE-CHEESE
E. SOUP & GRAIN	PROTEINS
PROTEINS	J. LOW-FAT DAIRY PROTEINS
F. LENTIL PROTEINS	K. DAIRY PROTEIN
	L. NON-VEGETARIAN
	ALTERNATIVE PROTEINS

RULE 5: • AVOID SNACKING.

RULE 6: • AVOID BEEF, TABLE SUGAR, WHITE FLOUR, GREASE, SALT, RED MEATS, DELICATESSEN LUNCHEON MEATS, AND ALL MEATS.

RULE 7: • RELAX WITH YOUR MEALS. CHEW EACH BITE SLOWLY.

RULE 8: • DRINK AT LEAST 6-8 GLASSES OF FLUID EACH DAY:
Two glasses of fresh fruit juice, one glass of fresh vegetable juice, and essentially five glasses of mineral-rich spring water. Herbal teas with raw honey (optional) are recommended.

RULE 9: • BE SURE YOUR FOOD IS HIGHLY PALATABLE.
Season your food with herbs from the Hi-Lite herb food kitchen. (See chapter on health food kitchen.)

HEAL YOUR NERVES

One of the more subtle but definitive benefits of the Maintenance Diet is the rejuvenating effect consistent balanced living nutrition has on your nerves. In fact, overstressed nerve roots, burned out glands and worn out cellular enzymes can be rehabilitated with such a program. The well-rounded Maintenance Diet provides the appropriate nutrients, especially essential amino acids, B vitamins, essential unsaturated fatty acids, minerals, trace elements, and whole grains to nourish your nerves. Keep in mind that your nerves are indispensable dynamic electrical wires. They carry messages from your environment back to your brain and carry messages to your body from your mind. A healthy vital nervous system is a must for optimal health. An alert sharp nervous system is a prerequisite for healing. A well functioning right-on-the-money nervous system is needed to enable you to prevent disease. All too commonly, your nerves are bad because they burn out from overwork and too much emotional stress. This leads to a gradual but continual loss in alertness, responsiveness, and vitality. This loss in function is usually compounded by the excessive wear and tear of unpredictable circumstantial daily emotional stress, environmental pollutants, and dietary toxemia. A thoroughly balanced, hi-enzyme maintenance regime provides a daily elixir of vital healthy nutrients. This keeps your nerves sharp and properly wired. *The healthier your nervous system, the better health you will experience.*

YOUR OPTIMAL DIET KEEPS YOUR NERVOUS SYSTEM YOUNG AND VITAL

Alice, a 34-year-old housewife, had her hands full all day long. She had devoted the best years of her life to raising her family in a loving, healing atmosphere. She was intuitively committed to natural breastfeeding. Alice came to see me because she hadn't had one menstrual period for the last 3½ years. During this period of time, there wasn't a single week when she wasn't either pregnant or breastfeeding. At the recent birth of her new son, David, she finally had to wean her 14-month-old baby daughter, Tracy. After four months of breastfeeding, little David weaned himself from Alice to the bottle. Alice felt relieved and so did the baby. Her milk was not rich enough to keep up with his needs. Right about this time Alice's hair began to fall out. She went to see her family physician, who said everything checked out just fine. He told her to maintain a balanced diet, get more protein, and she'd be o.k. He gave her a printed handout so full of meat and dairy products that it looked like a brochure from the cattlemen and dairy association. She decided it was time to get some nutritional advice.

"Doctor Meltzer, I just can't take it any more. There is no way I can keep up with these screaming children. How come no one ever told me what it was like to have a new baby to care for, one child at 18 months, and two older children who are constantly needing my time and attention? When my husband comes home after working all day, I'm exhausted, yet he expects me to be ready to get up for a big evening. He doesn't want to hear the children crying, so recently he's been coming home later and later. I don't have the time or the energy to take care of my family or myself any more. Can you help me?"

"Are you getting enough rest?"

"No. Even the nights I get four to six hours of sleep. I wake up exhausted."

"You seem to be under a lot of stress."

"I am. My relationship with my husband is strained because I do not have the desire to be a social butterfly or an active sexual partner. The little time I do have I need to spend alone to get myself together. And naturally our relationship is suffering. On top of it all, our financial hassles seem endless, and so does the rising inflation."

Alice had been in good health all of her life, and had never experienced any real weakness or fatigue until the last two years.

A complete physical and battery of lab tests were all normal. After a thorough examination, I concluded that she was not anemic, nor did she have diabetes or an underactive thyroid gland. There was no evidence of tuberculosis nor did she have any obvious signs of malnutrition. I asked her to keep track of her food intake for one week.

"Keep good records of your eating habits for the next seven days. Record when and what you eat for breakfast, lunch, and dinner each day. Meet me back in my office in a week with your meal schedule."

When I examined Alice's dietary patterns one week later, I found her meal schedule to be irregular. She would eat whatever she could whenever it was available. Her daily menu went something like this:

Breakfast: One bowl of cereal or two slices of toast and butter with eggs and sausages. And whatever soup or casserole was left over from the night before.

Lunch: Hamburger on a bun at MacDonald's. Raisins, bread snacks, and crackers with apricot marmalade.

Dinner: Beef or chicken, a smattering of lettuce, potatoes, rolls, and cheesecake for dessert.

Snacks consisted of milk, cookies, raisins, 7-Up, cokes, figs, and bread.

My analysis of her diet revealed it to be the usual: high in animal protein, high in fat, and high in nutrition-poor carbohydrates. It was rich in refined carbohydrates, concentrated sweet carbohydrates and starches, but low in true dietary fiber.

I informed Alice that her imbalanced diet could not sustain a high energy level.

"Packaged, processed food is wearing you down. You're living a slow death. Your diet lacks fresh, raw, live food, and as a result is Hi·Lite enzyme deficient. You need a wholesome, living, hi-enzyme, balanced maintenance regime to rehabilitate your system. The nutritional formula for correcting your condition is the Hi·Lite Hi-Enzyme Maintenance Diet.

"Alice, an optimal Maintenance Diet supplies the correct amount of natural, hi-enzyme fresh fruits, vegetables, fruit and vegetable juices. Are you in touch with what percentage of your diet is fresh, raw food, and what percentage is cooked, devitalized, fried and greasy? Your ratio is way out of balance. Fresh foods are badly needed in your diet. The proper ratio of fresh raw foods to cooked foods is fundamental to keeping your diet balanced to promote healing and prevent disease. This is the art of the Del Mar Diet. It will keep your body highly energized."

The typical American diet is anything but balanced. It usually contains a *ratio of from 2:1 and sometimes even 4:1 cooked food in favor of fresh raw food.* To verify the exact ratio you need only attend a Sunday brunch, a potluck, a buffet, a wedding reception, eat at a popular restaurant, or simply read the menu at a local diner to see the proportion of cooked food to raw food available. Too much cooked and processed food lowers the enzyme value in your diet. *The nutritional truth is that the best maintenance regimen has at least a 1:1 ratio or at least 50 percent fresh raw foods to cooked foods in your meals.*

Raw fruits and vegetables are high fiber foods. Appropriate dietary fiber is a major feature of a balanced Maintenance Diet. Dietary fiber is the roughage present in carbohydrates that are resistant to human digestive enzymes. *The chief sources of fiber, in addition to raw fruits and green vegetables, include whole grain breads, whole grain cereals, corn, the peel of a baked potato, and of course wheat bran and rice bran.* Dietary fiber leaves a high residue. It does its job as an intestinal broom to sweep the waste matter, poisons, and toxins out of your lower intestine.

Color also plays an important role in keeping your balanced Maintenance Diet together. Each and every high quality food speaks to us with a radiance and a beautiful complexion unique to its own self. The fresh vital *red colors of beets, tomatoes, radishes, and red cabbage* add visual extrasensory zest to your raw vegetable salads. The *red fruits — strawberries, apples, and cherries —* add decor and passion to the kaleidoscope of your diet. Deep *green leafy vegetables such as lettuce, spinach, zucchini, chard, and sprouts* are visually soothing and physiologically healing to your mind, body, and spirit. *Yellow fruits such as apricots, peaches, melons, and bananas* have a sweet and inviting glow. The balance in the color of your diet is conducive to your overall nutritional balance. Be sure to prepare your salad with a rainbow mixture of high quality fresh, living fruits and vegetables that complement each other in a balanced, aesthetic, harmonious way.

To overcome her long-term fatigue, I placed Alice directly on the Maintenance Diet. A typical day of eating on the Maintenance Diet was:

Breakfast:	(1)	Fresh watermelon juice (6 oz.), 15 minutes later
	(2)	**BASIC MELON SALAD** with cantaloupe, watermelon, and honeydew.
	(3)	1-2 slices 7-grain sprouted toast with natural unsalted peanut butter.
Lunch:	(1)	**LEAFY-GREEN CHLOROPHYLL SALAD**
	(2)	**COWBOY RANCH DRESSING**
	(3)	**MELTZER B.L.T. SANDWICH** (bread, lettuce, tomato)
	(4)	A bowl of vegetable-bean soup
Dinner:	(1)	Fresh carrot-celery-beet juice (8 oz.) 15 minutes later
	(2)	**SUPER SPROUT SALAD,**
	(3)	**LEMON-GARLIC DRESSING**
	(4)	**STEAMED GREEN VEGETABLE PLATTER** with broccoli and zucchini
	(5)	Soyburger on whole wheat bun

After three weeks on just the Maintenance Diet, Alice's fatigue began to disappear. Then I instructed her to spend seven days on the Cleansing Diet. I explained to her that were she to have any weakness, fatigue, or headaches with her Cleansing Diet she should add:

- 1½ Tbsp. of brewers yeast as needed every four hours to a glass of fresh grapefruit juice.

- A green vegetable broth each day to provide a plentiful supply of potassium to neutralize acid toxins.

I advised her to supplement her Maintenance Diet with 2 mg. of folic acid, 100 mcg. of vitamin B-12, a high-potency B-complex vitamin with each meal, 250 mg. of magnesium oxide once in the morning, and a chelated mineral supplement two times a day. She also took an all-purpose multi-vitamin three times a day.

After one week of cleansing, Alice then continued with the Hi·Lite Detoxification Diet. She then briskly followed with the Hi·Lite Maintenance Diet Plan. After six weeks from the start of the program, the strength returned to her body. She began to feel like her old self again. Within three months, Alice was busier than ever because her middle son was approaching the terrible two's. With the living, balanced, hi-enzyme Maintenance program, Alice found that she could handle the stress in her own life while participating fully in the joys of her family life.

WEEK 3 — THE MELTZER MAINTENANCE DIET: DAY 15
REVIVE IT: TRANSFUSE IT

Juice fast today in accordance with the seasonal laws of juice fasting. Refer to page 74 on **Day 8** on the Detoxification Diet.

JUICE FAST SCHEDULE

Spring:		Summer:	
7:00 a.m. —	orange or watermelon	7:00 a.m. —	watermelon
10:00 a.m. —	carrot	10:00 a.m. —	carrot
1:00 p.m. —	orange or watermelon	1:00 p.m. —	watermelon
4:00 p.m. —	carrot	4:00 p.m. —	carrot
7:00 p.m. —	orange or watermelon	7:00 p.m. —	watermelon
10:00 p.m. —	carrot-celery or carrot-celery-beet	10:00 p.m. —	carrot-celery or carrot-celery-beet
Autumn:*		**Winter:**	
7:00 a.m. —	apple	7:00 a.m. —	orange or grapefruit or pineapple
10:00 a.m. —	carrot		
1:00 p.m. —	apple	10:00 a.m. —	carrot
4:00 p.m. —	carrot	1:00 p.m. —	orange or grapefruit or pineapple
7:00 p.m. —	apple		
10:00 p.m. —	carrot-celery or carrot-celery-beet	4:00 p.m. —	carrot
		7:00 p.m. —	orange or grapefruit or pineapple
		10:00 p.m. —	carrot-celery or carrot-celery-beet

HI· LITE NUTRITIONAL MAINTENANCE BREAKFAST
(7:00·8:00 a.m.)

Spring:
(1) Papaya-pineapple juice (6 oz.)
   15 minutes later
(2) **SOUTH AMERICAN TROPICAL FRUIT SALAD**
   • Papaya, ½ cup
   • Pineapple, ½ cup
   • Banana, 1 medium
(3) Almonds (1 oz.)-Granola (2 oz.)
(4) Alfalfa sprouts (as much as you want)

Summer:
(1) Watermelon juice (6 oz.)
   15 minutes later
(2) **SUMMER MELON SALAD**
   • Cantaloupe, ½ medium
   • Watermelon, ½ cup
   • Honeydew, ½ cup
(3) Almonds (1 oz.)-Granola (2 oz.)
(4) Alfalfa sprouts (as much as you want)

Autumn:
(1) Apple juice (6 oz.)
   15 minutes later
(2) **WALDORFF APPLE SALAD AMBROSIA**
   • Pippin apple, ½ medium
   • Pear, ½ medium
   • Banana, 1 medium
(3) Almonds (1 oz.)-Granola (2 oz.)
(4) Alfalfa sprouts (as much as you want)

Winter:
(1) Orange juice (6 oz.)
   15 minutes later
(2) **WINTER CITRUS SALAD**
   • Orange, 1 medium
   • Pink grapefruit, ½ med.
   • Pineapple, ½ cup
(3) Almonds (1 oz.)-Granola (2 oz.)
(4) Alfalfa sprouts (as much as you want)

HI·LITE NUTRITIONAL MAINTENANCE LUNCHEON
(12:30·2:00 p.m.)

Lightweight
(1) **FRUIT SALAD SUPREME**
(2) ½ cup low-fat cottage cheese

Welterweight
(1) **GARDEN GREEN CHLOROPHYLL SALAD**
(2) KELP-FROM-THE-SEA DRESSING
(3) TERRIFIC TABOULI with 2 tsp. sunflower seeds in salad

Heavyweight
(1) **GARDEN GREEN CHLOROPHYLL SALAD**
(2) KELP-FROM-THE-SEA DRESSING
(3) THE PITA STUFF inside whole wheat pita bread
(4) Mixed vegetable soup

HI·LITE NUTRITIONAL MAINTENANCE DINNER
(5:30·7:00 p.m.)

(1) Fresh carrot, carrot-celery or carrot-celery-beet juice (8 oz.) *15 minutes later*
(2) **GARDEN PEA SALAD**
   • Chinese snow peas, 12
   • Romaine lettuce, 4 leaves
   • Green peas, 2 tbsp.
   • Green pepper, ½ large
   • Alfalfa sprouts, ½ cup
   • Tomato, ½ large
      • ONION-GARLIC DRESSING
      • Sesame or sunflower seeds, 2 tsp.
(3) Gourmet Vegetarian Dinner Night: **ZUCCHINI·BROCCOLI·RICE VEGETABLE CASSEROLE**

HI· LITE NUTRITIONAL MAINTENANCE BREAKFAST
(7:00-8:00 a.m.)

Spring:
(1) Orange juice (6 oz.)
   15 minutes later
(2) **ZESTY SPRING SALAD**
   • Pineapple, ½ cup
   • Banana, 1 medium
   • Strawberries, 5 large
(3) Seven-grain sprouted toast,
   1-2 slices with peanut butter
(4) Alfalfa sprouts (as much as
   you want)

Summer:
(1) Watermelon juice (6 oz.)
   15 minutes later
(2) **SUMMER MELON SALAD**
   • Cantaloupe, ½ medium
   • Watermelon, ½ cup
   • Honeydew, ½ cup
(3) Seven-grain sprouted toast,
   1-2 slices with peanut butter
(4) Alfalfa sprouts (as much as
   you want)

Autumn:
(1) Pear juice (6 oz.)
   15 minutes later
(2) **MIXED APPLE SALAD**
   • Pippin apple, ½ medium
   • MacIntosh apple, ½ medium
   • Golden Delicious apple,
     ½ med.
(3) Seven-grain sprouted toast,
   1-2 slices with peanut butter
(4) Alfalfa sprouts (as much as
   you want)

Winter:
(1) Orange juice (6 oz.)
   15 minutes later
(2) **ORANGE WONDERLAND
   SALAD**
   • Orange, ½ medium
   • Pineapple, ½ cup
   • Banana, ½ medium
(3) Seven-grain sprouted toast,
   1-2 slices with peanut butter
(4) Alfalfa sprouts (as much as
   you want)

HI·LITE NUTRITIONAL MAINTENANCE LUNCHEON
(12:30-2:00 p.m.)

Lightweight
(1) **SUPER SPROUT
   SALAD**
(2) LEMON-GARLIC
   DRESSING
(3) Raw or steamed
   carrots, peas,
   mushrooms and 2 tsp.
   sunflower seeds
   to salad

Welterweight
(1) **SUPER SPROUT
   SALAD**
(2) LEMON-GARLIC
   DRESSING
(3) PICES POTATO
   SALAD with 2 tsp.
   sunflower seeds

Heavyweight
(1) **SUPER SPROUT
   SALAD**
(2) LEMON-GARLIC
   DRESSING
(3) MID-EASTERN
   GARBANZO SPREAD
   with whole wheat
   pita bread

HI·LITE NUTRITIONAL MAINTENANCE DINNER
(5:30-7:00 p.m.)

(1) Fresh carrot, carrot-celery or carrot-celery-beet juice (8 oz.) *15 minutes later*
(2) **RAW MUSHROOM SALAD**
   • Romaine lettuce, 4 leaves
   • Sprouts, ½ cup
   • Tomato, ½ large
         • Mushrooms, 10 small or 4 large
         • Cucumber, six 1/8-inch slices
         • Celery, 1 stalk
       • LEMON-VINAIGRETTE DRESSING
         • Sesame or sunflower seeds, 2 tsp.
(3) Chinese Food Night: **VEGETARIAN CHOP SUEY**
   • Tofu
   • Chinese vegetables
   • Green vegetables
         • Mushrooms
         • Brown or wild rice

HI· LITE NUTRITIONAL MAINTENANCE BREAKFAST
(7:00-8:00 a.m.)

Spring:
(1) Papaya juice (6 oz.)
   15 minutes later
(2) **MANGO DAYBREAK DELIGHT**
   • Mango, ½ medium
   • Banana, ½ medium
   • Pineapple, ½ cup
(3) Whole grain toast with peanut butters, 1-2 slices
(4) Alfalfa sprouts (as much as you want)

Summer:
(1) Papaya juice (6 oz.)
   15 minutes later
(2) **CHERRY-FRIAR PLUM SALAD**
   • Cherries, 8
   • Friar plum, 1
   • Nectarine, 1 medium (or other variety of plum)
(3) Whole grain toast with peanut butter, 1-2 slices
(4) Alfalfa sprouts (as much as you want)

Autumn:
(1) Apple juice (6 oz.)
   15 minutes later
(2) **AUTUMN ENERGY SALAD**
   • Pippin apple, ½ medium
   • Papaya, ½ cup
   • Banana, 1 medium
(3) Whole grain toast with peanut butter, 1-2 slices
(4) Alfalfa sprouts (as much as you want)

Winter:
(1) Grapefruit juice (6 oz.)
   15 minutes later
(2) **PAPAYA PARADISE SALAD**
   • Orange, ½ medium
   • Papaya, ½ cup
   • Banana, 1 medium
(3) Whole grain toast with peanut butter, 1-2 slices
(4) Alfalfa sprouts (as much as (you want)

HI·LITE NUTRITIONAL MAINTENANCE LUNCHEON
(12:30-2:00 p.m.)

Lightweight
(1) **FRUIT SALAD SUPREME**
(2) ½ cup low-fat cottage cheese or ½ cup non-fat yogurt

Welterweight
(1) **COOL CUCUMBER SALAD**
(2) **AVOCADO GREEN DRESSING**
(3) **LANI'S LIMA-BEAN RICE SOUP**

Heavyweight
(1) **COOL CUCUMBER SALAD**
(2) **AVOCADO GREEN DRESSING**
(3) **TOFU BURGER** on whole wheat bun

HI·LITE NUTRITIONAL MAINTENANCE DINNER
(5:30-7:00)

(1) Fresh carrot, carrot-celery or carrot-celery-beet juice (8 oz.) *15 minutes later*
(2) **SUPER SPROUT SALAD**
   • Bean sprouts, all you want
   • Alfalfa sprouts, all you want
   • Sunflower seed, sprouts, all you want

   • Romaine lettuce, 4 leaves
   • Tomato, ½ large
   • Red onion, ¼ cup

   • HERBAL VINAIGRETTE DRESSING
   • Sesame or sunflower seeds, 2 tsp.
(3) Cleansing Night: **BAKED POTATO** with **CLEANSING CHILI SAUCE** and **MIXED VEGETABLE SOUP** or **STEAMED VEGETABLE PLATTER**

HI·LITE NUTRITIONAL MAINTENANCE BREAKFAST
(7:00-8:00 p.m.)

Spring:
(1) Papaya-pineapple juice (6 oz.)
15 minutes later
(2) **CHERRY SUPREME SALAD**
  • Cherries, 8
  • Peach, 1 medium
  • Banana, 1 medium
(3) Mixed nuts, 1-3 oz.
(almonds, cashews, walnuts)
Raisins or other dried fruits
can be added to the salad:
For example: 1 tsp. raisins
1 fig or 1 date
(4) Alfalfa sprouts (optional)

Summer:
(1) Papaya juice (6 oz.)
15 minutes later
(2) **APRICOT SUNSHINE SALAD**
  • Apricots, 3 medium
  • Peach, 1 medium
  • Plum, 1 medium (or 8
cherries or 1 cup seedless
grapes)
(3) Mixed nuts, 1-3 oz.
Raisins or other dried fruits
can be added to the salad.
(4) Alfalfa sprouts (optional)

Autumn:
(1) Apple Juice (6 oz.)
15 minutes later
(2) **PEACEFUL PEAR SALAD**
  • Pear, 1 medium
  • Papaya, 1 cup
  • Banana, 1 medium
(3) Mixed Nuts, 1-3 oz.
Raisins or other dried fruits
can be added to the salad
(4) Alfalfa sprouts (optional)

Winter:
(1) Orange Juice (6 oz.)
15 minutes later
(2) **PINK GRAPEFRUIT WINTER
SALAD**
  • Pink grapefruit, ½ medium
  • Orange, ½ medium
  • Banana, 1 medium
(3) Mixed nuts, 1-3 oz.
Raisins or other dried fruits
can be added to the salad
(4) Alfalfa sprouts (optional)

HI·LITE NUTRITIONAL MAINTENANCE LUNCHEON
(12:30-2:00 p.m.)

Lightweight
(1) **MEXICAN CABBAGE
SALAD**
(2) LEMON-GARLIC
DRESSING
(3) ½ cup steamed
carrots, ½ cup
steamed peas, 8
medium mushrooms,
2 tsp. sunflower seeds
in salad

Welterweight
(1) **MEXICAN CABBAGE
SALAD**
(2) LEMON-GARLIC
DRESSING
(3) **MIGHTY MUSHROOM
CARROT-ONION
SOUP** with 1-2 tsp.
sunflower seeds added
to salad.

Heavyweight
(1) **MEXICAN CABBAGE
SALAD**
(2) LEMON-GARLIC
DRESSING
(3) **LUSCIOUS LENTIL
SOUP** with 1-2 slices
pita bread

HI·LITE NUTRITIONAL MAINTENANCE DINNER
(5:30-7:00 p.m.)

(1) Fresh carrot, carrot-celery or carrot-celery-beet juice (8 oz.) *15 minutes later*
(2) **SPICE-OF-LIFE SPINACH SALAD**
  • Spinach, 4 leaves
  • Romaine lettuce, 2-4 leaves
  • Tomato, ½ large

  • Alfalfa sprouts, ½ cup
  • Red onion, ¼ medium
  • Celery, 1 stalk

  • ONION-GARLIC DRESSING
  • Sesame or sunflower seeds, 2 tsp.
(3) Italian Night: **EGGPLANT PARMESAN,** with whole grain garlic bread.

HI·LITE NUTRITIONAL MAINTENANCE BREAKFAST
(7:00-8:00 a.m.)

Spring:
(1) Papaya juice (6 oz.)
15 minutes later
(2) **GRAPE DELIGHT SALAD**
  • Seedless green grapes, 1 cup
  • Red grapes, ½ cup
(3) Whole-grain sprouted toast with peanut or almond butter, 1-2 slices
(4) Alfalfa sprouts (as much as you want)

Summer:
(1) Papaya juice (6 oz.)
15 minutes later
(2) **HAWAIIAN FRUIT SALAD**
  • Papaya, ½ cup
  • Mango, ½ medium
  • Pineapple, ½ cup
(3) Whole-grain sprouted toast with peanut or almond butter, 1-2 slices
(4) Alfalfa sprouts (as much as you want)

Autumn:
(1) Pear juice (6 oz.)
15 minutes later
(2) **WALDORF APPLE SALAD AMBROSIA**
  • Pippin apple, 1 medium
  • Pear, ½ medium
  • Banana, 1 medium
(3) Whole-grain sprouted toast with peanut or almond butter, 1-2 slices
(4) Alfalfa sprouts (as much as you want)

Winter:
(1) Orange juice (6 oz.)
15 minutes later
(2) **SOUTH AMERICAN TROPICAL FRUIT SALAD**
  • Pineapple, ½ cup
  • Papaya, ½ cup
  • Banana, 1 medium
(3) Whole-grain sprouted toast with peanut or almond buter, 1-2 slices
(4) Alfalfa sprouts (as much as you want)

HI·LITE NUTRITIONAL MAINTENANCE LUNCHEON
(12:30-2:00 p.m.)

Lightweight
(1) **FRUIT SALAD SUPREME**
(2) ½ cup low-fat cottage cheese or non-fat yogurt.

Welterweight
(1) **AVOCADO-TOMATO GRANDE SALAD**
(2) RED CAYENE DRESSING
(3) **LUSCIOUS LENTIL SOUP**

Heavyweight
(1) **AVOCADO-TOMATO GRANDE SALAD**
(2) RED CAYENE DRESSING
(3) SOY BURGER on whole wheat bun

HI·LITE NUTRITIONAL MAINTENANCE DINNER
(5:30-7:00 p.m.)

(1) Fresh carrot, carrot-celery or carrot-celery-beet juice (8 oz.) *15 minutes later*
(2) **GARDEN-GREEN CHLOROPHYLL SALAD**
  • Romaine lettuce, 2-4 leaves
  • Spinach, 4 leaves
  • Alfalfa sprouts, ½ cup
  • Tomato, ½ large
  • Swiss chard, 1-2 leaves
  • Parsley, 1 tbsp.
  • Red onion, ¼ medium
  • Carrot, 1 medium
    • LEMON-GARLIC DRESSING
    • Sesame or sunflower seeds, 2 tsp.
(3) Mexican Food Night: **ORGANIC TOSTADO**

HI·LITE NUTRITIONAL MAINTENANCE BREAKFAST
(7:00-8:00 a.m.)

Spring:
(1) Orange juice (6 oz.)
   15 minutes later
(2) **SOUTH AMERICAN TROPICAL FRUIT SALAD**
   • Papaya, ½ cup
   • Banana, 1 medium
   • Pineapple, ½ cup
(3) Almonds (½ oz.) with 7-grain cereal or oatmeal (½ bowl)
(4) Alfalfa sprouts (as much as you want)

Summer:
(1) Papaya juice (6 oz.)
   15 minutes later
(2) **NECTARINE-PEACH SALAD**
   • Nectarine, 1 medium
   • Peach, 1 medium
   • Cherries, 8
(3) Almonds (½ oz.) with 7-grain cereal or oatmeal (½ bowl)
(4) Alfalfa sprouts (as much as you want)

Autumn:
(1) Apple juice (6 oz.)
   15 minutes later
(2) **AUTUMN ENERGY SALAD**
   • Pippin apple, ½ medium
   • Papaya, ½ cup
   • Banana, 1 medium
(3) Almonds (½ oz.) with 7-grain cereal or oatmeal (½ bowl)
(4) Alfalfa sprouts (as much as you want)

Winter:
(1) Orange juice (6 oz.)
   15 minutes later
(2) **PINK GRAPEFRUIT WINTER SALAD**
   • Pink grapefruit, ½ medium
   • Orange, ½ medium
   • Banana, 1 medium
(3) Almonds (½ oz.) with 7-grain cereal or oatmeal (½ bowl)
(4) Alfalfa sprouts (as much as you want)

HI·LITE NUTRITIONAL MAINTENANCE LUNCHEON
(12:30-2:00 p.m.)

Lightweight
(1) **RADIANT RADISH SALAD**
(2) HERBAL ITALIAN DRESSING
(3) Add raw carrots, peas, cauliflower and 2 tsp. sunflower seeds to salad

Welterweight
(1) **RADIANT RADISH SALAD**
(2) HERBAL ITALIAN DRESSING
(3) OLD WORLD POTATO-LEEK SOUP ½ cup cottage cheese with the salad

Heavyweight
(1) **RADIANT RADISH SALAD**
(2) HERBAL ITALIAN DRESSING
(3) SPICY SPLIT PEA SOUP with 1-2 slices pita bread

HI·LITE NUTRITIONAL MAINTENANCE DINNER
(5:30-7:00 p.m.)

(1) Fresh carrot, carrot-celery or carrot-celery-beet juice (8 oz.) *15 minutes later*
(2) **JICAMA-BEET TREAT**
   • Jicama, ½ cup
   • Raw grated beet, ½ medium
   • Carrot, 1 small
   • Romaine lettuce, 4 leaves
   • Tomato, ½ large
   • Alfalfa sprouts, ½ cup
      • KELP-FROM-THE-SEA DRESSING
   • Sesame or sunflower seeds, 2 tsp.
(3) **SOYBURGER** on whole wheat bun
(4) **MIXED VEGETABLE SOUP** (optional)

PLEASE NOTE that you can use a variety of fresh salads and complete protein exchange combinations. You can vary your entrees and make your diet an interesting, exciting, total experience.

7: MAINTENANCE DIET RECIPES

The following pages will give you the specific food preparation tips to fully allow the Maintenance Diet to go to work for you. The recipes are categorized according to the standard food groups of the Maintenance Diet.

FOOD GROUPS 1a and 2a: Fresh Fruit and Raw Vegetable Juices

Your fruit juice and raw vegetable choices are the same as for the Cleansing and Detox Diets. Carrot-celery-parsley or fresh tomato juice are legitimate additional choices for your daily vegetable juice. Mellow herbal teas are recommended. Nut milks, elixirs, and tonics are also acceptable to maintain the proper nutrient-rich fluid intake of your Maintenance Diet.

Almond-Sesame Milk

1 cup almonds (soaked overnight in 2 cups water)	1 Tbsp. honey to taste (or molasses)
½ cup sesame seeds	1½ Tbsp. Brewers yeast
2-3 cups water	1 tsp. vanilla (optional) or use ¼ vanilla bean and blend with nuts

Retain the overnight water and blend almonds and sesame seeds with water on high speed for 2-3 minutes. Strain and return nut milk to blender. Then add honey, Brewers yeast, and vanilla. Almond-sesame pulp can be used in nut loafs or bread. Carob powder (1 Tbsp.) can also be added for variety. Substitute 1 banana in place of honey for less calories. Garnish with a sprinkle of cinnamon.

This recipe is especially beneficial for the pregnant or nursing woman or for children who need to increase their protein and calcium intake. The molasses adds nutritional iron when needed.

Ginger Fizz

1-inch piece fresh peeled ginger
Juice of ½ lemon per glass,
    to taste

Honey to taste
Sparkling mineral water

Finely chop or grate ginger. Boil 15 minutes in one cup water. Strain and divide liquid into 2 tall glasses. Squeeze ½ lemon into each glass. Fill to top of glass with sparkling mineral water. Garnish with bee pollen sprinkled on top.

Specialty Drinks:

Sunday Brunch Delight

Fresh orange juice
Fresh pineapple juice

White champagne

Mix equal amounts of orange and pineapple juice. Use half juice and half champagne. Enjoy!

Summertime Fruit-Tea Punch

8 cups boiling water
4 cinnamon sticks, broken
1 Tbsp. whole cloves
A few dashes nutmeg

4 teabags, herbal
Juice of 2 lemons
2 Tbsp. honey, to taste
24 ounces pineapple juice

Add one of the following:

24 ounces fresh grapefruit juice or 24 ounces fresh orange juice.

Bring water to a boil in a large stainless steel or enamel saucepan. Add spices and teabags. Remove teabags after three minutes of steeping. Let remainder of spices simmer for about twenty minutes. Add lemon juice and the two remaining juices. Bring just to a boil, leave on lowest heat to keep warm. For a larger crowd, add another 3 cups of fresh pineapple juice.

Makes about 40 servings.

Avocado Apertif

1 medium size avocado
1 large cucumber
Juice of 1 lemon
½ cup parsley, chopped

1 Tbsp. sesame oil
2 cups crushed ice
Lemon slices or cucumber peel

Peel avocado and cucumber, chop in chunks and place in blender. Add parsley, lemon, and oil and blend until smooth. Add the crushed ice and blend together again. Strain into large glasses. Garnish with lemon slices or cucumber peel. Makes four servings.

FOOD GROUP 1: Hi·Lite Fresh Fruit Salad Supremes

Fall, winter, spring, and summer options guide your seasonal selections. Consult Cleansing Diet, page 21.

FOOD GROUP 2: Hi·Lite Leafy Green Chlorophyll Salads

The choices are the same as the Cleansing and Detoxification Diet raw vegetable salads.

FOOD GROUP 3: Complete Protein Fruit Exchanges

A **Hi·Lite Fruit Salad Supreme** with any **one** of the following will make breakfast into a complete protein meal:

    (1) 1 oz. almonds with 2 oz. granola
    (2) 1-2 Tbsp. nut butter with 2 oz. granola
    (3) 1-2 slices sprouted 7-grain bread with 1-2 Tbsp. nut butter
    (4) 1 oz. almonds with half a bowl 7-grain cereal, oatmeal, millet, bran, cream-of-rye or cream-of-wheat cereal
    (5) 1-3 oz. mixed nuts

FOOD GROUP 4: Lightweight Luncheon Complete Protein Exchanges

FOOD GROUP 4a: Lightweight Fruit Luncheon Complete Protein Exchange

A **Hi·Lite Fruit Salad Supreme** with any **one** of the following will make a lightweight fruit luncheon into a balance of raw food and complete protein:

    (1) ½ cup low-fat cottage cheese
    (2) ½ cup non-fat yogurt
    (3) 1-3 oz. nuts and seeds
    (4) **Meltzer Lightweight Fruit Smoothie** (Take any Fruit Salad Supreme using appropriate seasonal fruits and blend together with 1-2 Tbsp. brewers yeast and 1 tsp. bee pollen.)

FOOD GROUP 4b: Lightweight Vegetable Luncheon Complete Protein Exchange

A **Hi•Lite Leafy-Green Chlorophyll Salad** plus any **one** of the following will make a lightweight luncheon into a balance of raw food and complete protein:

(1) Raw carrots, peas, mushrooms, and 2 tsp. sunflower seeds added to salad.

(2) Raw carrots, peas, cauliflower, and 2 tsp. sunflower seeds added to salad.

(3) ½ cup steamed carrots, ½ cup steamed peas, 8 medium mushrooms, and 2 tsp. sunflower seeds added to salad.

(4) 1 cup steamed green vegetables of the season with 2 tsp. sunflower seeds added to raw sprouted salad.

FOOD GROUP 5: Welterweight Luncheon Complete Protein Exchanges

A **Hi•Lite Leafy-Green Chlorophyll Salad** * plus any **one** of the following will make your welterweight luncheon into a balance of raw food and complete protein:

(1) **Terrific Tabouli**
(See Detoxification Recipes)

(2) **Tofu Salad**

Tofu, 8 oz.	1 Tbsp. brewers yeast
1 stalk finely chopped celery	½ tsp. cumin
1-2 chopped green onions	½ tsp. dill
or ¼-½ chopped red onion	½ tsp. tumeric
1 medium tomato, sliced in wedges	½ tsp. Dr. Bronners seasoning

Mash tofu with a fork and mix with balance of ingredients except tomato. Refrigerate one hour to blend flavors. Serve on a bed of lettuce leaves. Top with sprouts and arrange tomato wedges around. Garnish with paprika. Soy spread can replace Tofu Salad.

Soy Spread

1½ cup cooked soybeans	1 clove garlic, minced
1 Tbsp. oil	1 tsp. basil
¼ cup onion, chopped	½ tsp. oregano
¼ cup celery, chopped	1 small tomato, chopped

Saute all ingredients in oil except soybeans. Meanwhile, grind soybeans in blender or food processor. Blend soybean mixture with sauteed mixture. Great on whole grain breads.

(3) **Lani's Lima Bean-Rice Soup**
(See Detoxification Recipes, page 97).

(4) **Bean Vegetable Soup**
(See Detoxification Recipes, page 97).

(5) **Spicy Split Pea Soup**

½ cup split peas	1-2 stalks celery, chopped
1 bay leaf	5 mushrooms, sliced
1 clove garlic, pressed	½-1 tsp. curry (optional)
1 red onion, chopped	1 Tbsp. parsley
1-2 sliced carrots	1 tsp. dill

Bring 2 cups water to a boil in covered kettle. Add peas and bay leaf. Turn down heat and simmer 30 minutes. Add balance of ingredients and simmer 15 minutes longer or until peas are done. To make a creamy soup, you can put part or all of it in the blender, then return to pan.

---

* With 2 tsp. sunflower seeds in salad.

(6) **Mighty Mushroom and Carrot-Onion Soup**

2 doz. mushrooms, sliced	1-2 stalks celery, sliced
2-3 carrots, sliced in rounds	1 tsp. dill
1-2 red onions, chopped	Vegetable cube (1 low-sodium from
1 bay leaf	Switzerland) or desired seasonings

Bring 3 cups water to a boil. Add ingredients and cover. Simmer until carrots are tender.

(7) **Luscious Lentil Soup** with 2 tsp. sunflower seeds in salad
(See Detoxification Recipes, page 97).

(8) **Pisces Potato Salad** (eggless)

4 medium Russet potatoes, or red or new potatoes	1 Tbsp. lemon juice
	1 tsp. dill
2 stalks celery, chopped	½ medium green pepper, chopped
1 red onion, chopped	2 Tbsp. parsley
2 Tbsp. cold-pressed safflower oil	1 tsp. mustard, prepared without
Eggless mayonnaise	preservatives
½ medium dill pickle, chopped	¼ tsp. kelp powder
(without preservatives) (optional)	Paprika (sprinkle on top before
	serving)

Cut potatoes in half lengthwise and steam. Cool and chop in large chunks. Add balance of ingredients and mix well. Chill several hours or overnight. Garnish with paprika. Serves 2.

(9) **Old World Potato-Leek Soup**

2-3 large potatoes, diced
2 leeks, sliced
2 medium carrots, sliced in
  thick chunks
2 cloves garlic
1 bay leaf
1 cup fresh peas

8-12 mushrooms, sliced
1 pinch cayenne
1 tsp. dill
Several springs fresh parsley
  (or 1 Tbsp. dried)
Paprika, sprinkled on top

Cook first 5 ingredients in 4 cups water until almost done (test carrots with a fork). Place half of the mixture in the blender (cool slightly first) and cream. Return to pot and add balance of ingredients. Cook over low heat 10 more minutes or until peas are tender. Sprinkle with paprika before serving.

(10) **Wholly Guacamole** (avocado salad)
(See Cleansing Recipes, page 64).

(11) **Vegetarian Taco** (fresh raw or steamed vegetables inside a warm corn tortilla).

(12) **Avocado Sandwich** on 2 slices of sprouted 7-grain bread.

(13) **The Pita Stuff** (avocado, tomato, sprouts, and onions inside whole wheat pita bread).

(14) **Lake Taco** (Guacamole Taco) — Wholly Guacamole on corn tortilla or whole wheat chapati without cheese.

FOOD GROUP 6: Heavyweight Luncheon Complete Protein Exchanges

A **Hi•Lite Leafy-Green Chlorophyll Salad** plus any **one** of the following will make your heavyweight luncheon into a balance of raw food and complete protein:

(1) **Avocado Sandwich** on 2 slices of sprouted 7-grain bread and mixed vegetable soup.

(2) **Avocado Sandwich** with choice of vegetable, bean, or pea soup.

(3) **The Pita Stuff** (avocado, tomato, sprouts, and onions inside whole wheat pita bread) and mixed vegetable soup.

(4) **Luscious Lentil Soup** — with 2-3 slices sprouted 7-grain bread (See Detoxification Recipes).

(5) **Mid-Eastern Garbanzo Spread** (Hommus) with whole wheat pita bread

2 cups cooked garbanzo beans, drained (save liquid)
1 Tbsp. sesame oil
Juice of 1 large lemon
1 clove garlic, minced
½-1 tsp. cumin

¼ cup parsley, finely minced
¼ cup scallions, finely minced
1/8 tsp. cayenne
¼ cup sesame seeds or more (optional)

Blend garbanzo beans, oil and lemon juice in blender or food processor. When smooth add remaining ingredients. Add garbanzo bean liquid to achieve desired consistency. Chill. Serve as a raw vegetable or cracker dip or on whole wheat breads.

(6) **Terrific Tabouli** stuffed inside whole wheat pita bread (See Detoxification Recipes, page 92).

(7) **Wholly Guacamole** with vegetable bean soup (See Cleansing Recipes).

(8) **Lake Taco** (Guacamole Taco) — Wholly Guacamole on corn tortilla or whole wheat chapati without cheese, with a bowl of mixed vegetable or bean soup.

(9) **Romona's Quesadillas —** with or without mixed vegetable soup.

Whole wheat flour tortillas or corn tortillas
Grated rennetless cheese or mozzarella (about ¼ cup per tortilla)

Salsa (or chopped tomatoes)
Green onions, chopped

Place tortilla in heated pan. Set cheese on half of tortilla. Top cheese with salsa and green onions, to taste. Cook over medium heat until cheese melts and tortilla is warm. Fold tortilla in half and serve.

(10) **Feeling Great Filafel**

4 cups cooked garbanzo beans (chickpeas) or 2 cups soaked 1½ hrs., boiled until very soft
3 medium cloves garlic, crushed
½ cup celery, finely minced
½ cup scallions, finely minced
½ tsp. ground cumin
½ tsp. tumeric

¼ tsp. cayenne
Dash of black pepper
3 Tbsp. tahini
3 Tbsp. flour or fine bread crumbs
Olive oil or sesame oil for sauteeing patties

Mash the well-cooked garbanzo beans well. Combine with rest of ingredients. Chill well. Flour hands and make the mixture into patties 3-4 inches in diameter. Roll in flour or bread crumbs. Saute in olive oil until golden and serve.

Serving suggestion: Serve with garden salad of diced cucumbers, tomatoes, and peppers with pita bread to complement this Middle-Eastern feast.

(11) **Lani's Lima Bean-Rice Soup** (See Detoxification Recipes) — with 1-2 slices sprouted 7-grain or whole wheat pita bread.

(12) **Vege-Burger:** Mushroom, soy, lentil, garbanzo, or tofu burger without bread with vegetable bean soup. (See soy-burger recipe.)

(13) **Vege-Burger** with whole wheat bun.

(14) **Spicy Split Pea Soup** (See Maintenance Recipes) with 1-2 slices sprouted 7-grain or whole wheat pita bread.

(15) **Bean Vegetable Soup** (See Detoxification Recipes) with 1-2 slices sprouted 7-grain or whole wheat pita bread.

(16) **Mighty Mushroom-Carrot-Onion Soup** (See Maintenance Recipes) with 1-2 slices sprouted 7-grain or whole wheat pita bread.

FOOD GROUP 7: Complete Dinner Protein Exchanges

A **Fresh Leafy Chlorophyll Salad** with any one of the following will make your dinner into a balance of raw food and complete protein:

FOOD GROUP 7a: Complete Cleansing Exchanges

These are self-explanatory. See Maintenance Diet, Group 7a, page 109.

FOOD GROUP 7b: Complete Tofu Exchanges

(1) 4 oz. **Scrambled Tofu** (See Detoxification Recipes), 4 medium mushrooms, sauteed.

(2) 4 oz. **Scrambled Tofu,** ½ cup wild rice, brown rice, or wild rice-brown rice mixture.

(3) Vegetarian chop suey with 4 oz. **Scrambled Tofu**, ½ cup wild-brown rice, plus mung bean sprouts, Chinese cabbage, mushrooms, celery, onions (See Detoxification Recipes, page 95).

(4) Tofu-vegetable-mushroom-rice casserole with 4 oz. tofu, green vegetables, mushrooms, and brown rice.

(5) Tofu-mushrooms-**Rico Vegie Rice Casserole** with 4 oz. tofu and sauteed mushrooms (See Detoxification Recipes, page 95).

(6) 2 oz. tofu with mixed vegetable-rice soup (See Detoxification Recipes).

(7) **Pisces Potato Salad** (eggless) (See Detoxification Recipes) with 2-3 oz. Scrambled Tofu and steamed green vegetables.

(8) **Tofu Burger**

1 lb. tofu, sliced in squares	Cumin
Kelp	Cayenne
Dill	

For each tofu slice, place in lightly oiled skillet and sprinkle with above seasonings on both sides. Cook on medium-high heat 4 minutes. Turn and cook an additional 3 minutes.

FOOD GROUP 7c: Complete Soybean Exchanges

(1) **Soybean-brown rice-vegetable casserole** (See Maintenance Recipes): ½ cup cooked soybeans, with ½ cup cooked brown rice or wild rice, vegetable casserole.

(2) **Soyburger** (or Sesame-Soyburger)

Soak overnight:

1 cup dry whole soybeans
2 cups water

Drain and cook at a gentle boil in 4 cups water with 1 bay leaf. When the soybeans turn dark they're done (approx. 8 hrs.). Yields 2½ cups cooked beans. Remove bay leaf, drain and mash with a fork and add:

¾ cup sesame meal (sesame seeds can be ground in blender)
1 medium yellow onion, finely chopped (or several green onions)
1 large garlic clove, pressed
½ small green pepper, finely chopped
2 cups mushrooms, finely chopped
½ stalk (⅓ cup) celery, finely chopped

Mix together well and add:

1 Tbsp. lemon juice
2 Tbsp. tamari
3 Tbsp. oil

Mix well and form into patties. Place on oiled baking dish and bake at 350° for 30 minutes or until they turn brown. Makes six 6-oz. patties (wt. before cooking).

Serve with green salad and one of the following:
(1) One steamed green vegetable
(2) Sprouted whole wheat bun, lettuce, sprouts, and salsa
(3) 1 oz. cheese melted on burger for vegetarian cheeseburger — with one steamed green vegetable.

(3) **Soyburger on whole grain bun**

(4) **Soy-cheeseburger** (Place 1 oz. of raw, rennetless, or low-fat cheese over soyburger)

(5) **Soy-cheeseburger with whole grain bun**

(6) ½ cup soy grits with ½ cup cooked brown rice (See Detoxification Recipes).

(7) One Soyburger made into soyballs with whole grain noodle vegetarian spaghetti (Dr. Barney's favorite — See Maintenance Pasta Recipe, page 134.).

FOOD GROUP 7d: Complete Bean Exchanges

(1) Organic Tostadas

To correctly prepare the corn tortillas so that they are crisp, they must be prepared in a small amount of oil. To achieve maximum crispness, place just enough **safflower oil** to cover bottom of frying pan, then heat oil to a medium heat. Do not allow oil to smoke. Place corn tortilla in oil and cook on both sides, only seconds at a time, turning tortillas twice, or until crisp (a very short amount of time).

Remove from pan.
Place on paper towel to cool and remove excess oil.

Or use purchased tortillas or chapatis and heat in oven.

Prepare:

Crisp tortillas	Diced onions
Beans (heated right before serving)	Avocados, sliced
	Grated cheese
Shredded lettuce	Salsa picante
Diced tomatoes	

(2) **Feeling Great Filafel** (See Maintenance Recipes, page 129).

(3) **Hommus Lebanese Dip** (See Maintenance Recipes, page 123).

(4) **Beans** (mung beans, aduki beans, lima beans, kidney beans, pinto beans) with brown or wild rice, ½ cup each.

How to Cook Beans

One cup dry beans makes approximately 2½ cups cooked.

Beans (1 cup dry)		Water	Cooking Time
Black	soaked overnight	4 cups	2-3 hours
Black-eyed peas	unsoaked	3 cups	1 hour
Garbanzos	soaked overnight	3 cups	2-3 hours
Great Northern	soaked overnight	3 cups	1 hour
Kidney and red	unsoaked	3 cups	90 minutes
Kidney and red	soaked 1 hour	3 cups	60 minutes
Lentils	unsoaked	3 cups	60-90 minutes
Lentils	soaked 1 hour	3 cups	45 minutes
Lima	unsoaked	3 cups	90 minutes
Lima	soaked 1 hour	3 cups	45 minutes
Navy	unsoaked	3 cups	90 minutes
Navy	soaked 1 hour	3 cups	60 minutes
Pinto	unsoaked	3 cups	2-2½ hours
Pinto, split	unsoaked	2 cups	45 minutes
Soybeans	soaked overnight	4 cups	3 hours
Split peas	unsoaked	3 cups	45 minutes

Suggested seasonings: 1 Tbsp. lemon juice when beans are tender, chopped carrots, celery added last ½ hr. Dill, celery seed, garlic, vegetable bouillion cube.

FOOD GROUP 7e: Complete Soup and Grain Exchanges

(1) **Lima bean-vegetable soup** (See Detoxification Recipes), with 1-2 slices whole grain bread.

(2) **Lima bean-vegetable soup** (See Detoxification Recipes), with brown rice.

(3) **Split Pea Soup** (See Maintenance Recipes, page 133), with ½ cup brown or wild rice.

(4) **Split Pea Soup** (See Mainenance Recipes, page 133), with 1-2 slices whole grain or whole wheat pita bread.

(5) **Minestrone-bean-vegetable Soup,** with ½ cup brown rice.

Refer to Detoxification Recipe, making the following modifications:

Use: 1 cup red kidney beans
      1 cup pinto beans   instead of lima beans
      ½ cup garbanzo beans

Follow same directions except rinse and soak the beans overnight or for specified time (see How to Cook Beans). Cook beans separately with bay leaf and enough water until tender. Combine the beans, vegetables, etc. as in Detox Recipe.

(6) **Minestrone-bean-vegetable Soup,** with 1-2 slices whole grain bread.

(7) Whole grain spaghetti artichoke, spinach, or soy noodles with natural tomato sauce and creamy mushroom soup.

Pasta

In a large kettle bring 3-4 quarts of water to rolling boil. Add 1 Tbsp. oil. Add pasta, stir with a fork to separate and boil approximately 10-12 minutes. Test pasta by removing some from water, cooling under cool water and tasting to see if it's tender. When done, remove from heat, drain off hot water, rinse pasta with warm water and serve. Whole grain pastas usually have a heavier consistency. Add natural tomato sauce to flavor.

Creamy Mushroom Soup

½ cup cashews, blended in	1 tsp. dill
4 cups water	1 cube vegetable bouillion or Tamari
1 yellow onion, chopped	1 carrot, chopped
1 Tbsp. oil	1-2 large leaves chard, chopped
15 medium mushrooms, chopped	1-2 stalks celery, chopped

Saute onion in oil. Add mushrooms, celery, carrot, and chard. Stir. Add cashew milk and seasonings and simmer on low until thick and creamy. Do not boil.

(8) Whole grain spaghetti noodles, with natural tomato sauce (see above), mixed with Scrambled Tofu and served with the following soup:

Cream of Beet Soup

4 red potatoes, chopped	1 pinch cayenne	1 Tbsp. miso
1 yellow onion, chopped	½ tsp. kelp	
1 carrot, chopped	1 Tbsp. dill	
2 small zucchini, chopped	1 stalk celery, chopped	
2 beets, chopped	2 cloves garlic, minced	

Cook all ingredients, except miso in 4 cups water. When vegetables are tender blend all to smooth consistency, adding more water if needed. Add miso, cover and cook on low heat for 5-10 minutes.

FOOD GROUP 7f: Complete Lentil Exchanges

(1) **Lentil-Mixed Vegetable Soup** (See Detoxification Recipes), with raw or sauteed mushrooms.

(2) **Lentil-mushroom-vegetable Casserole**

1 cup zucchini, sliced	¼ cup onion, chopped
1 cup broccoli, broken in flowerets	2 Tbsp. parsley, chopped
1 cup carrots, sliced	1 cup cooked lentils
2 tomatoes, chopped	1 cup cold water

Steam lightly zucchini, broccoli, and carrots. Place alternate layers of steamed vegetables and lentil mixture in casserole. Heat in 325° oven for 15 minutes.

(3) **Lentil-sesame or Lentil-cashew Nut Roast**

3 cups lentils (med. soft puree)	1 tsp. sage
1½ cups raw nuts (chopped cashews or walnuts)	½ tsp. celery seed
½ cup ground sunflower seeds or sesame seeds	1 Tbsp. tamari
1 Tbsp. onion, minced	4 Tbsp. sunflower oil
½ cup raw oatmeal or soft bread crumbs (3 slices)	¼ tsp. ground pepper

Mix well. Bake in oiled loaf pan for one hour at 350°. Serve with a mushroom gravy.

(4) **Lentil Soup** (See Detoxification Recipes, page 97), with 1-2 slices whole grain or whole wheat pita bread.

(5) **Lentil Soup** (See Detoxification Recipes, page 97), with ½ cup brown rice or millet.

(6) **Lentil Burger**

Soak 1 cup dry lentils in 2 cups water for 1 hour. Drain and cook at a gentle boil in 3 cups water with 1 bay leaf. When lentils are tender they're done. Remove bay leaf, drain, and mash with a fork and add:

¾ cup sesame meal (sesame seeds can be ground in blender)
1 medium yellow onion, finely chopped (or several green onions)
1 large garlic clove, pressed
½ small green pepper, finely chopped
2 cups finely chopped mushrooms
½ stalk (⅓ cup) celery, finely chopped

Mix together well and add:

1 Tbsp. lemon juice
2 Tbsp. tamari
3 Tbsp. safflower oil

Mix well and form into patties. Place on oiled baking dish and bake at 350° for 30 minutes or until they turn brown. Makes six 6-oz. patties. Serve on whole wheat bun.

FOOD GROUP 7g: Complete Pea Exchanges

(1) Steamed carrots, steamed peas, 1 baked potato with 2 tsp. sesame seeds added to raw vegetable salad.

(2) Vegetable casserole with steamed peas, mushrooms, and steamed greens with ½ cup brown rice and sesame seeds (2 tsp.) added to raw salad.

(3) Steamed peas, ½ cup, **Marinated Mixed-Bean Salad**, ¼ cup, 2 tsp. sesame seeds added to raw vegetable salad.

Marinated Mixed-Bean Salad

½ cup dry garbanzo beans	½ medium red onion, or as desired
½ cup dry red kidney beans	½ medium green pepper, chopped
1 cup steamed and chopped green beans	1 stalk celery, chopped

Cook garbanzo and kidney beans until tender (See section on How to Cook Beans under Maintenance Diet). Add balance of ingredients and cover with marinade.

Marinade

¼ cup honey	1 Tbsp. parsley
½ cup oil	1 tsp. basil
2 Tbsp. apple cider vinegar	

Chill several hours.

FOOD GROUP 7h: Complete Vegetable-Grain Casseroles

(1) **Stuffed Bell Peppers**

2 cups cooked brown rice, buckwheat, groats or millet	½ cup parsley, chopped
8 bell peppers	Pinch of cayenne
1 large yellow onion, chopped	Tomato sauce or chopped tomatoes
2 Tbsp. safflower oil	Other chopped vegetables of choice, i.e., celery, carrots, broccoli, chopped finely.
3 cloves garlic crushed	

Cut off tops of peppers and remove seeds. Steam shells for 8 minutes. Saute onions in oil until tender. Add garlic, parsley and vegetables and cook 5 minutes longer. Add rice, tomatoes or sauce and blend together. Fill shells and arrange upright in a baking dish. Top with grated cheese or serve with yeast gravy. Bake 350°, 30 minutes. For additional texture and protein, add 8 oz. of chopped tofu to rice mixture.

(2) **June's Indian Vegetable Curry** with brown rice or millet

1 medium onion, chopped	3 cloves garlic, crushed
2 Tbsp. safflower oil	1 tsp. curry
1 cup peas	2 bay leaves, crumbled
1 cauliflower, separated	½ tsp. grated ginger
3 carrots, sliced and quartered	1/8 tsp. cayenne (optional, spicy)
1 medium eggplant, cut in 1" squares	½ cup water
2 tomatoes, chopped	

In a large saucepan heat oil and saute onion until clear. Add cauliflowerets, carrots, eggplant, peas, and tomatoes. Season with garlic, curry, ginger, bay leaves and cayenne. Pour in water. Cover and simmer until the vegetables are of desired tenderness. Serve in its own liquid. Brown rice or millet would be a compatible side dish. Other vegetable combinations: cabbage, potato, peas and tomato: tomato, peas, spinach and squash.

(3) **Balinese Tempeh in Mushroom Sauce**

1 lb. tempeh	½ tsp. ginger root, fresh grated
3-4 large tomatoes	1 red or yellow onion, chopped
1 clove garlic, minced	6-12 mushrooms, sliced
	Cumin
	Dill

Blend the tomatoes with garlic and ginger. Heat in saucepan with the onion and mushrooms. Cover and simmer 15-20 minutes, then turn heat to lowest setting. If tempeh is still frozen, place block on cookie sheet and brush all over with tomato sauce. Sprinkle with cumin and dill. Proceed to bake at 350° until it is soft enough to cut into ½" cubes. Brush again with tomato sauce and bake 20-30 minutes until lightly browned. Mix tempeh with tomato/mushroom sauce and serve over rice or whole grain pasta.

FOOD GROUP 7i: Vegetable-Cheese Casseroles

(1) **Eggplant-Rice-Cheese Casserole**

1 eggplant, peeled and diced	2 tomatoes, chopped
1 cup zucchini, sliced	¼ cup onion, chopped
1 cup broccoli, broken in flowerets	2 Tbsp. parsley, chopped
1 cup carrots, sliced	½ cup brown rice, raw
	1 cup cold water
	Grated cheese

Steam lightly eggplant, zucchini, broccoli, and carrots. Cook remaining ingredients with the brown rice for 40 minutes. Place alternate layers of steamed vegetables and rice mixture in casserole. Then add grated cheese to cover and heat in 325° oven for 15 minutes.

(2) **Eggplant Parmesan**

Saute:
1 onion, chopped
1 clove garlic, pressed in safflower oil

Add:

4 tomatoes (liquified in blender)	½ tsp. thyme
1 tsp. basil	Pinch rosemary
1 tsp. oregano	1 tsp. tamari (or more to taste)
	1 tsp. kelp

Heat and thicken with 1 tsp. arrowroot dissolved in as little water as possible. Cook and stir, adding more arrowroot if necessary to thicken. Add 1-1½ cups sliced mushrooms and 1 stalk celery, chopped. Wash 1 large eggplant and slice in ½" rounds. Brush top of each slice with olive oil and sprinkle with basil and oregano. Broil until browned. Turn over and repeat with oil and herbs. Brown. Place eggplant slices in baking dish and top with tomato sauce and grated cheese. Sprinkle with paprika. Bake uncovered at 350° for 15-20 minutes. Serve with tossed green salad and rice and one steamed green vegetable.

(3) **Zucchini-Rice-Cheese Casserole** (See Rico Vegie-Rice Casserole — Detoxification Recipes — adding cheese on top).

(4) **Green Vegetable-Rice-Cheese Casserole**

(5) **Whole Grain Lasagna or Carol's Eggplant Lasagne**

1 small eggplant, diced ¼" thick	16 oz. Italian tomato sauce
½ onion, chopped	6-8 oz. tofu, broken up into cottage
½ green pepper, chopped	cheese texture
5 medium mushrooms, chopped	8 oz. mozzarella cheese, grated
1 clove garlic, pressed	¼ cup parmesan cheese
¼ cup oil	

Broil eggplant brushed with sesame oil until softened and browned. Set aside on paper towels. Saute onion, green pepper, mushrooms. Spoon Italian sauce to cover bottom of baking dish. Layer eggplant and sauteed vegetable mixture with tofu, then mozzarella cheese, followed by tomato sauce and top with parmesan cheese. Bake at 350° for ½ hour. Serves 4.

For Whole Grain Lasagna substitute whole grain lasagne noodles for eggplant slices.

(6) **Vegetarian Pita Pizza**

Italian tomato sauce (or use	Mushrooms, sliced
thinly sliced tomatoes sprinkled	Onions, chopped
with basil and oregano	Grated cheese or crumbled tofu
Zucchini, sliced	

On pita bread spread sauce or place tomatoes. Cover with other ingredients, placing cheese or tofu on top. Bake 10-15 minutes at 350° or until cheese melts.

FOOD GROUP 7j: Low-Fat Dairy Exchanges

(Low-fat yogurt, farmer's cheese, ricotta cheese, skim milk or mozzarella cheese, buttermilk, hoop cheese, low-fat cottage cheese)

(1) Steamed green vegetables, 1 baked potato and one serving from above.

(2) **Minestrone-Mixed Vegetable Bean Soup** with one low-fat dairy exchange.

(3) **Eggplant Parmesan** (See Maintenance Recipes, page 138), with ricotta cheese.

(4) **Ratatoulli** (with low-fat dairy products)

1 eggplant, peeled and sliced	1 clove garlic, minced
3 zucchini, sliced	2 large tomatoes, halved, cut into
2 green peppers, diced	½ inch strips, and drained
1 onion, thinly sliced	½ tsp. oregano
	¼ tsp. ground pepper

Combine all the ingredients in a large, heavy pot. Cook, covered, over low heat for 20 minutes. Cook, uncovered, 15 minutes more over moderate heat, stirring with a wooden spoon to prevent scorching. Can be baked in a 350° oven for one hour as an alternative method of cooking. Top with grated cheese and melt under broiler. Serves 4.

(5) **Vegetarian Pizza** (See Maintenance Recipes, page 138), with skim milk, farmer's or mozzarella cheese.

FOOD GROUP 7k: Dairy Exchanges

(Raw or rennetless cheddar, colby, jack cheese)

(1) **June's Cheese Enchiladas** (with ½ cup brown rice)

FILLING: 12 corn tortillas

3 yellow onions, sliced and quartered	8 oz. grated raw jack or cheddar cheese
3 Tbsp. safflower oil	10 mushrooms, chopped
4 cloves garlic, crushed	6 green onions, sliced
8 oz. ricotta cheese	

Heat oil in a large skillet. Saute onions and garlic until golden. Turn off heat and add remaining ingredients. Mix well; set aside.

SAUCE: (For dipping tortillas and baking enchiladas)

6 oz. tomato paste
3 cups hot water
1 clove garlic, crushed
1 tsp. ground cumin

2 tsp. chile powder
2 tsp. tamari
2 green chiles (baked and skinned),
   mashed

Combine all ingredients in a shallow bowl and mix well. Follow directions for Spinach Enchiladas. Before baking, lightly garnish top with grated cheese, sliced green onions and diced radishes.

(2) **Romona's Quesadilla**, with vegetable soup.

(3) **Romona's Quesadilla**, with beans.

(4) **Spinach Enchiladas**

3-4 dried pasilla chilies, remove seeds (be careful not to touch your eyes after
   you have handled chilies)
1 tsp. oregano
1 doz. corn tortillas
12 oz. grated mozarella or mild cheddar cheese
2 medium red onions, chopped
1-2 medium green pepper's, chopped
Chopped green onions
1 bunch spinach, fresh leaves

Pour 2 cups boiling water over chilies, cover and let set 1 hour. Place in blender with oregano. Cook over low heat. Saute onion in skillet, using as little oil as possible. Add green pepper and spinach. Saute until spinach is wilted. Heat tortillas on hot grill using as little oil as possible. Dip in sauce. Place mixture of spinach in center, add a little sauce, grated and chopped. Roll up. Put in shallow baking dish. Cover with remaining sauce, garnish with cheese and green onions and bake at 350° uncovered for 30 minutes.

FOOD GROUP 8: Maintenance Salad Dressings

Select any **Herbal Salad Dressing** from the Cleansing and Detoxification Recipes. Additional salad dressings on the Maintenance Diet include:

(1) **Herbal Yogurt Dressing**

8 oz. plain, low-fat yogurt
1 tsp. dill
Juice of 1 lemon

1 tsp. parsley
1 green onion, chopped (or chives)
1 tsp. tamari

Mix and chill one hour before serving.

(2) **Cowboy Ranch Dressing**

8 oz. low-fat cottage cheese
¼ cup parsley, chopped
¼ cup scallions, chopped

1 clove garlic, minced
Buttermilk

Put cottage cheese, parsley, scallions and garlic in blender or food processor. Blend until fairly smooth. Add buttermilk to attain desired consistency.

(3) **The Original "I Street" Yeast Gravy**

½ cup brewers yeast
¾ cup rice cream (rice flour)
1 onion, chopped

¼ cup or less tamari
¼ cup oil
4 cups water or to desired
consistency

Saute onion in oil. Add yeast, tamari and oil and stir. Add water slowly. Simmer over low heat, stirring frequently.

(4) **Salsa Picante**

1 large tomato
1 or 2 chilies (Use fresh green hot chilies, usually about 2½" long, found with the yellow chilies in produce department. Use 1 or 2 of these chilies to 1 tomato, depending on how hot you like your salsa.)

Place under the broiler until the chilies and tomato pop. You may have to turn the chilies and tomato to the other side. Heated chilies and tomatoes are MAS SALOBROSO (very HOT). Blend in blender to your basic salsa. After blending, you may add oregano and diced onion.

FOOD GROUP 9: Maintenance Diet Desserts

(1) **Crispy Apple Treat**

6 medium pippin apples, unpeeled,
cored and sliced
Juice from 1 lemon
1 Tbsp. cinnamon (or more
to taste)

¾ cup walnuts, chopped
1-2 Tbsp. honey
1-2 Tbsp. safflower oil
1 tsp. nutmeg, ground
1 tsp. cloves, ground

Place apples in pie dish. Sprinkle with lemon juice. In separate pan add safflower oil and honey. Add walnuts and spices. Place over apples and bake 350° for 20-30 minutes.

(2) **Tasty Toasted Almond Fruit Pie Crust**

1 cup toasted almonds, ground
½ cup oat flour (rolled oats put
in blender)
1 tsp. honey

⅓ cup coconut, grated, fresh
or dried
Safflower oil
1 tsp. honey

Combine safflower oil and honey. Mix in other ingredients. Press into 8" pie plate. Cook 350° for 10 minutes. Fill with your favorite raw fruit pie filling.

(3) **Crusty Wheat Germ Fruit Pie**

1¼ cups wheat germ, raw or toasted	¼ cup oil
¼ cup bran	2 Tbsp. honey
	⅓ cup coconut

Mix well. Press into 8" pie plate. Use raw or bake 10 minutes at 350°.

Fantastic Fruit Filling

2 cups fresh fruit (use a juicy seasonal fruit)	1 tsp. cinnamon
Juice from 1 lemon	1 Tbsp. honey
	1 stick agar-agar

Soak agar in 1¼ cup water. Heat and stir constantly until liquified. Blend fruit with ¼ cup water. Add lemon, honey and cinnamon. Taste and adjust spices. Turn blender on low and add agar to fruit. Pour into cooled pie crust. Garnish with your choice of fruit, nuts, seeds, coconut, or raisins. Chill until firm.

A GLOSSARY OF NUTRITIONAL FOOD TERMS

AGAR: A sea weed used like gelatin for making fruit.

ARROWROOT FLOUR: Used as a thickening agent instead of corn starch or flour.

CAROB FLOUR: Used to replace chocolate in desserts.

KELP: Dried and ground seaweed which can be used as a seasoning instead of salt.

MISO: Soybean paste produced by enzymatic fermentation and aging of soybeans. Add at the very end of cooking so as not to destroy the enzymes.

RICE BRAN SYRUP: A liquid yeast composed of the B-complex vitamins, especially rich in B3.

SMOOTHIE: A "fruit shake" made by blending fruits and juices.

SPIRULINA: A powdered sea algae high in protein and B-12.

TAHINI: Made from hulled sesame seeds ground into a butter much like peanut butter.

TAMARI: A soy sauce made without sugar and chemicals. Can be diluted and used in place of salt to add flavor to dressings.

TEMPEH: Tempeh is a prepared soybean product made from the fermentation of cracked soybeans. It is easily digested and is a rich source of vitamin B-12.

TOFU: Soybean curd or soy cheese. Tofu can be purchased in health food stores and prepared by scrambling with onions, mushrooms, and tamari or saute the tofu with the vegetables.

8: THE DEL MAR PERMANENT WEIGHT LOSS PROGRAM

The Del Mar permanent weight loss program can't be beat for safe, reliable, long-term weight loss. It is a Life·time Eat Right Diet to get in shape and stay that way. It works for folks who need to lose 7 pounds or those who need to lose 107.

The program is simple and Light. The diet is easy to prepare and is satisfying to your palate. Step-by-step you eat well and get great results in a short period of time. Your weight comes down smoothly. All the while, the permanent weight loss program teaches you the self-discipline and self-control of sensible, proper eating habits. This keeps you looking lean, trim, and fit year after year.

Remember, any way you cut the cheesecake, permanent weight loss calls for a smart diet coupled with sound eating habits. A vigorous 15-20 minute daily workout and a positive self-image hold the program together. Continuous, steady weight reduction requires motivation and consistency. With the guidelines and operating manual of the Del Mar Diet, you can make it happen.

The Del Mar Diet is a fantastic way to lighten a burdensome load. How much can you expect to take off and how fast can you lose it?

Bear in mind that you have a choice with the dynamic Del Mar Diet. You can lose it gradually or swiftly. It is up to you.

Plan I: The Gradual Approach

The more gradual routine is to go with the basic 21 Day Del Mar Diet (see Chapter 1) and follow it up with its seasonal rhythm method:

Basic 21 Day Program: WEEK 1: *Cleansing*
WEEK 2: *Detoxification*
WEEK 3: *Maintenance*

In this fashion you lose 10-15 lbs. in the first three weeks. Then, the rhythm method takes over. By juice fasting one day a week, cleansing right before the seasonal change, detoxifying at the mid-seasonal juncture, and watching to stay within the boundaries of nutritional maintenance, you will lose an additional 8-12 lbs. each month.

The rule of thumb is that with the basic plan you lose at least 25-50 lbs. in the first three months. It all happens very naturally. You lose until you are just right. With the original Del Mar Diet plan, you can be sure to reduce down to your lean muscle mass and stay that way. Keep in mind that when you use a standard maintenance diet for your weight loss plan, limit yourself to two meals a day. Choose either breakfast and dinner or lunch and dinner. Avoid snacking. This kind of weight loss is very legitimate and very respectable.

SUMMARY: PLAN I

Week 1:	Cleansing	
Week 2:	Detoxification	Lose 10-15 lbs. first three weeks.
Week 3:	Maintenance	
Follow the Del Mar		
rhythm method.		Then, drop 8-12 lbs./month.
	Gradual 50 lb. weight loss: 4-6 months	

Follow the rhythm method of the Del Mar Diet until you are within 25-30 lbs. of your desired weight. Then you can go back to the basic 21-day plan and safely lose another 10-15 lbs. in three weeks. With only 10-15 lbs. left, you can finish up with the seasonal plan of the Del Mar Diet to get your job done.

EXAMPLE 1: Mrs. K. Z. — 5'5" — Age 29 — Starting weight: 147 lbs.
                                                              Goal: 121 lbs.

End Week 1	Wt. 140
End Week 2	Wt. 136
End Week 3	Wt. 133
Loss of	14 lbs.
1 month later	Wt. 125
2 months later	Wt. 121
3 months later	Wt. 121

Plan II: Lose It Swiftly

In the rapid weight-loss program, the first week of the 21-day plan shifts gears upwards to quicken the pace. On the first two days you prepare to juice fast by eating only fresh fruits and raw vegetables. You follow this up with a 5-day juice fast. This completes your first week. When you do it right and you continue to exercise each day, you can easily lose 7-10 lbs. in the first week.

Rapid Weight Loss	WEEK 1:	*Juice Fasting*
21 Day Del Mar Diet:	WEEK 2:	*Cleansing*
	WEEK 3:	*Detoxification*

Week 2 consists of your basic Del Mar Cleansing Diet. Dropping another 5-7 lbs. is common. In Week 3, on the Detox Diet, be sure to limit yourself to one slice of bread at lunchtime. Also, leave off the high-energy pickups at 10:30 and 3:30 unless your energy level needs a shot in the arm. Figure that on detox you take off another 3-4 lbs. by the end of the week. One other option is to eat only two meals a day on the Detox Diet and leave out either lunch or breakfast. This would guarantee you to be an additional 5-7 lbs. lighter at the end of the detox week.

By the end of the 21-day rapid weight loss plan, you lose anywhere from 15-21 lbs. You then have two choices. You can continue to lose weight gradually or more rapidly. By following up with the standard Del Mar rhythm method, you will lose, on the average, another 8-12 lbs. per month. By going on to the Del Mar Take·Charge·Keep·Trim Diet, you lose 12-20 lbs. each month. Both methods provide enough complete protein and natural carbohydrate to keep your system fueled while you burn up unwanted fat.

SUMMARY: PLAN II

Week 1:	Juice Fast	
Week 2:	Cleansing	Lose 15-21 lbs.
Week 3:	Detoxification	
Go to standard rhythm method		Go to Take·Charge·Keep·Trim Diet
Lose 8-12 lbs./month		Lose 12-20 lbs./month
Lose 50 lbs. in 3½-5 months		Lose 50 lbs. in 2½-3 months

The Del Mar Diet Breeds Success

One additional strategy for your permanent weight loss plan is to remain on your Take·Charge·Keep·Trim Diet for only three weeks at a time. After 21 days you can then return to three more weeks of the basic 21 day Del Mar Diet or the rapid 21 day weight loss plan. You can continue with this unique 21 day on and 21 day off program and safely reach your desired weight.

For example, Mr. S.K., Age 46, 5'11", weighed 231 lbs. when he started the Del Mar Diet. His desired weight was 165. Here is how he did it.

21 Day Rapid Weight Loss Plan:	Lost 21 lbs.
21 Day Take·Charge·Keep·Trim:	Lost 12 lbs.
21 Day Rapid Weight Loss Plan:	Lost 18 lbs.
21 Day Take·Charge·Keep·Trim:	Lost 12 lbs.
	Down to 169 lbs.

In four 21-day cycles Mr. S.K. lost 62 lbs. He then went to the standard Del Mar rhythm method and within two weeks was at 165. He is still at that current weight.

So there you have it. Your most prudent plan is to alternate between periods of active and then slower loss. Depending on your weight and your condition, be assured that one of your above weight-loss routines will work. The unique nutritional strategy of the Del Mar Diet is your breakthrough to success regardless of past failures. The result is permanent weight loss and a new lease on life. You feel better, and you own a strong energy level.

Your Metabolism Counts

You see, the only way to permanently lose weight is to rejuvenate your metabolism. When your metabolism breaks down, it is very difficult to lose weight. The yo-yo effect of gaining and losing, then gaining and dieting eventually burns out your metabolism. In fact, to keep the weight off and prevent getting fat again calls for a very sound metabolism. Here is the punch and the power of the Del Mar Diet. The natural healing talents of its rhythm method fixes the worn and torn out metabolism that often plagues the dieter. In fact, a prudent low-calorie weight-loss program without cleansing, detoxifying, and flushing out the poisons from your system cannot and will not bring your metabolism back to life. A lethargic metabolism needs a shot in the arm. The natural internal purification from the Del Mar Diet is the answer. Daily exercise and stress reduction also help.

RULES FOR PERMANENT WEIGHT LOSS PROGRAM

Follow these simple rules to get your desired result:

I. THE DO'S:

1. Eat the right foods in the spirit of moderation.

2. Practice prudent undereating.

3. Earn your meals with hard work or physical exercise before eating.

4. Eat your meals at regular intervals.

5. Completely relax when you eat.

6. Enjoy your food. Keep your mental attitude positive.

7. Substitute intimate conversation, good company, and laughter for over-indulgence.

8. Eat only when you are hungry.

9. Eat exactly what is prescribed.

10. Get in at least one 15-20 minute workout daily, compatible with your current level of fitness. Do this within the first waking hour of each day.

11. Monitor your weight weekly.

II. THE DON'TS

1. Avoid snacking, nibbling, tasting, and raiding the freezer. Drink a mild herbal tea, natural mineral waters with lime, or your potassium vegetable broth* during meals to arrest your appetite. When you give in or lose it, eat only carrot or celery sticks between meals.

2. Do not overeat.

3. Do not become a victim of nervous eating habits.

4. Avoid binging on cheese, crackers, ice cream, desserts, fruits, nuts, or sweets.

5. Avoid snacking while you are cooking.

6. Avoid eating the last helping just so it won't go to waste.

7. Avoid eating or drinking while standing, walking, driving, or watching television.

8. Avoid eating when you are emotionally upset, anxious, bored, uptight, depressed, fatigued, or irritable.

9. Prepare your salads with the Cleansing Diet salad recipes without oil, mayonnaise, or other rich dressings.

10. Eat your vegetables and brown rice without butter, margarine, or fats.

Remember, overeating is a psychological substitute for love and affection. Eat well for good health. When you are not getting the results you want on this Del Mar Diet, get some professional help and re-align your emotional support systems at home and at work. Then try it again until you succeed.

DIET STRATEGY FOR THE 21 DAY RAPID WEIGHT LOSS PLAN
WEEK 1: JUICE FASTING

Juice fasting enhances the efficiency of your metabolic machinery. After a good 5-day juice fast you have a lot more energy when you come off the fast. Two days on fresh fruits and vegetables are necessary to prepare you for the 5-day juice fast — liquid only diet.

BLUEPRINT FOR DAY 1 AND 2

Early Morning

Good Morning!

15-20 minutes of aerobic exercise, deep breathing, and invigorating hydrotherapy, followed by:

FRUITARIAN BREAKFAST (7:00 — 8:00 a.m.)
(1) Fresh fruit juice in season (6 oz). *15 minutes later:*
(2) **MELTZER FRUIT SALAD SUPREME***
with 2-3 fresh seasonal fruits (total 1½ cups)
(3) Alfalfa sprouts (optional)
  • Nutritional supplements

Mid-day

Sunshine, relax your mind and body, followed by:

FRUITARIAN LUNCHEON (12:30 — 2:00 p.m.)
(1) Fresh fruit juice in season (6 oz.) *15 minutes later:*
(2) **MELTZER FRUIT SALAD SURPEME***
with 2-3 fresh seasonal fruits (total 1½ cups)
(3) Alfalfa sprouts (optional)
  • Nutritional supplements

Evening

15 minutes of relaxation and/or meditation, followed by:

VEGETARIAN DINNER (5:30 — 7:00 p.m.)
(1) Fresh carrot, carrot-celery, or carrot-celery-beet juice (8 oz.), *15 minutes later:*
(2) **HI · LITE LEAFY GREEN CHLOROPHYLL SALAD:****
Raw sprouted garden-crisp vegetables with romaine lettuce, tomato, and 3 select fresh, raw, green vegetables, with your choice of **HERBAL SALAD DRESSING.**
(3) **STEAMED VEGETABLE COMBINATION**
(a platter of 2-3 steamed vegetables) — or
BROCCOLI-MIXED GREENS VEGETABLE SOUP
  • Nutritional supplements

---

*See page 21
**See page 22

BLUEPRINT FOR DAYS 3 TO 7

Follow the juice fast instructions as per page 69. Remember to take the nutritional supplements prescribed for the Cleansing Diet. Keep in mind that juice fasting is a natural body cleanser. When solid food intake is halted, your body can begin to catch up with itself. Within 36 hours of beginning this highly spirited liquid-only diet, your body's natural radar system searches out impurities and toxins.

Regular juice fasting is a powerful detoxifying agent. Within 2-3 days toxins may start breaking out. You may be bothered by skin eruptions, foul body odors from under your arm or from your sweat, foul stools, or bad breath. You can slow down the detox process by getting a little additional protein. Put 1 ½ Tbsp. of brewers yeast and, if necessary, 1 tsp. of bee pollen into your juices. Do not fret. Sooner or later the dirt swept under the carpet has to be dealt with. Now is the time. Keep in mind that juice fasting is a reliable and valid self-healing discipline. As a rule of thumb, for every mile you can run you can safely juice fast 1 day. Many who can't run 5 miles do well juice fasting 5 days. Consult your physician before starting the 5 day juice fast.

TIPS FOR FEELING TOPS WHILE FASTING

TIP NO. 1: Fasting is a time for soul-searching. It is a marvelous opportunity to spend quiet time with nature. Be sure to take it easy.

TIP NO. 2: Juice fast because you believe in it.

TIP NO. 3: Continue to have at least one vigorous workout each day while juice fasting.

TIP NO. 4: Meditate or pray for at least 15 minutes twice a day while juice fasting. Sunrise and sunset are your best times to recharge your mind.

TIP NO. 5: Be certain to get a full night's rest.

TIP NO. 6: Take the nutritional supplements prescribed in the Cleansing Diet.

TIP NO. 7: Do not take an enema unless you have gone three days without a regular bowel movement.

TIPS ON HOW TO BREAK THE FAST

TIP NO. 1: Do not break the juice fast until you have first exercised and meditated. When you meditate focus on your most personal goals.

TIP NO. 2: Break a juice fast with fresh fruit. Watermelon is the fruit of choice. When watermelon is out of season, papaya, apple, or banana is preferable, in that order.

A common danger is that many a hard-earned, well-disciplined fasting program is ended in an Italian restaurant with pizza-pie, lasagna, or with Mexican foods. On Day 8 of your rapid weight loss plan, the day you are breaking your juice fast, first exercise and have your morning fruit juice before your morning meditation. Wait until your mind is clear. Then eat ½ cup from one of the recommended fruits on the Cleansing diet Breakfast. Wait 15 minutes and then have a bowl (1½ cups) of fresh fruit without any nuts, seeds, granola, toast, cereal, or dairy products. Resume your regular cleansing diet, but substitute your breakfast for your lunch and your lunch for your dinner on that first day. Then go forward with your Cleansing Diet. Bear in mind that when you get to the Take·Charge·Keep·Trim maintenance plan, juice fast one day a week.

WEEK 2: THE CLEANSING DIET

The guidelines and rules for your second week are the same as for the basic Cleansing Diet (page 15). Breakfast, lunch, and dinner options do not change. Nutritional supplements also remain the same.

WEEK 3: THE DETOXIFICATION DIET

Consult the blueprint, guidelines, and rules for Detox (page 65). Variations are in amounts only. Be certain not to overeat. At lunchtime restrict yourself to one slice of bread. Eliminate the 10:30 and 3:30 pickups unless you need to raise your energy level. Follow up the Rapid 21 Day Plan with the Take·Charge·Keep·Trim Diet.

THE TAKE · CHARGE · KEEP · TRIM DIET

The Take·Charge·Keep·Trim Diet is a low-fat diet. It has substantial carbohydrates and enough complete protein to keep you going.

There is no doubt about its safety and effectiveness. The diet is simple and basic. You don't have to be hassled by dramatic calorie-counting. Eat what is prescribed and follow the rules. You will lose 3-5 lbs. a week on this diet.

BLUEPRINT FOR THE TAKE·CHARGE·KEEP·TRIM DIET

Early Morning
Good Morning!
15-20 minutes of aerobic exercise, deep breathing, and invigorating hydrotherapy, followed by:
THE TAKE·CHARGE·KEEP·TRIM BREAKFAST (7:00-8:00 a.m.)
(1) Fresh fruit juice in season (6 oz.) *15 minutes later:*
(2) **HI·LITE FRUIT SALAD SUPREME***
with 2-3 fresh seasonal fruits (1½ cups) and
 • ½ cup low-fat cottage cheese, or 7-10 almonds
  • Nutritional supplements

Mid-morning
Herbal cleansing teas

Mid-day
Sunshine, relax your mind and body, followed by:
THE TAKE·CHARGE·KEEP·TRIM LUNCHEON (12:30-2:00 p.m.) with two options:

Option A:
(1) Fresh carrot or tomato juice (6 oz.) *15 minutes later:*
(2) **A HI·LITE LEAFY-GREEN CHLOROPHYLL SALAD****
Raw sprouted garden-crisp vegetables with romaine lettuce, tomato, and 3 select fresh, raw, green vegetables, with your choice of **HERBAL SALAD DRESSING** and ½ tsp. of sunflower or sesame seeds.
(3) One slice of whole-grain bread to be chosen from:
 • sprouted wheat bread   • corn tortilla
 • sprouted seven-grain bread   • whole wheat pita bread
 • chapati
(4) Two days a week you can add a cup of mixed vegetable or vegetable bean soup.

Option B
(1) Fresh fruit juice in season (6 oz.) *15 minutes later:*
(2) **HI·LITE FRUIT SALAD SUPREME***
with 2-3 fresh seasonal fruits (1½ cups) and
 • ½ cup low-fat cottage cheese
  • Nutritional supplements

Mid-afternoon
Herbal cleansing tea

Evening
15 minutes of relaxation and/or meditation, followed by:
THE TAKE·CHARGE·KEEP·TRIM BREAKFAST (5:30-7:00 p.m.)
(1) Fresh carrot, carrot-celery, or carrot-celery-beet juice (8 oz.) *15 minutes later:*
(2) **HI·LITE SPROUTED GARDEN-FRESH SALAD**
with your choice of **HERBAL SALAD DRESSING**
(3) **STEAMED VEGETABLE COMBINATION** (a platter of 1-2 steamed vegetables — OR 1 cup of **MIXED VEGETABLE SOUP**
(4) Choose one of the following complex carbohydrates:
 • ½ cup brown rice   • 1 corn on the cob
 • 1 medium baked potato   • 1 baked yam or squash
 • ½ cup millet
(5) One serving of complete protein every other day. Choose from:
 • 3-4 oz. tofu   • 4 oz. fish
 • 2-3 oz. low-fat dairy products • 4 oz. lean turkey
 • 2-3 oz. dried beans   • 4 oz. lean chicken
  • Nutritional supplements

After Dinner
Cleansing herbal tea

*See page 21
**See page 22

GUIDELINES FOR THE
TAKE·CHARGE·KEEP·TRIM DIET
FOODS ALLOWED ON THE TAKE·CHARGE·KEEP·TRIM DIET

Seasonal Fresh Fruits and Fruit Juices	yes	All fresh fruits in season. Avoid sweetened, frozen, canned, or packaged fruits. No dried fruits. The bottom line is one **HI·LITE FRESH FRUIT SALAD SUPREME** daily.
Fresh Vegetables and Raw Vegetable Juices	yes	All fresh raw vegetables can be included. Avoid frozen, canned, wilted, salted, or oiled vegetables.
Sprouts	yes	Living sprouts add life·force to the diet.
Nuts	yes	Almonds, in the amount of 7-10, can be eaten with your breakfast meal. Walnuts, cashews, or other nuts can be substituted for almonds.
Seeds	yes	½ tsp. sunflower seeds or sesame seeds is quality protein to be added to your luncheon.
Complex Carbohydrates and Whole Grains	yes	1 slice of whole-grain bread at lunch. 1 serving of complex carbohydrate at dinner.
Beverages	yes	Corresponding seasonal fruit juices and vegetable juices. Herbal teas, mineral waters, and natural water to the tune of 6-8 glasses of fluid a day.
Legumes	yes	As a protein option.
Dairy Products	yes	Low-fat cottage cheese or non-fat yogurt at breakfast. Low-fat dairy as a protein option every other evening.
Fish or Fowl	yes	As a non-vegetarian protein option every other evening. Limit to 4 oz. per serving.
Meat	no	Not advised for the Take·Charge Diet.

RULES FOR THE
TAKE·CHARGE·KEEP·TRIM DIET

Follow these simple rules and you will be rewarded mentally and physically.

RULE NO. 1: EAT AT LEAST 2 MEALS.

RULE NO. 2: BREAKFAST BETWEEN 7:00-8:00 A.M. FOR 30 MINUTES.

RULE NO. 3: LUNCH BETWEEN 12:30-2:00 P.M. FOR 30 MINUTES.

RULE NO. 4: DINE BETWEEN 5:30-7:00 P.M. Allow at least 30 minutes and up to 90 minutes.

RULE NO. 5: AVOID SNACKING.

RULE NO. 6: DRINK 6-8 GLASSES OF FLUID EACH DAY. Between meals drink only herbal teas and water.

RULE NO. 7: SEASON YOUR FOODS WELL WITH YOUR FAVORITE HERBS AND SPICES. AVOID SALT.

RULE NO. 8: DO NOT EAT ANY SWEETS. AVOID DESSERTS AND CANDIES. AVOID CAKES, PIES, COOKIES, JAMS, OR CHOCOLATE.

RULE NO. 9: DO NOT EAT HI-FAT DAIRY PRODUCTS.

RULE NO. 10: RESTRICT YOUR ALCOHOL INTAKE TO 8 OZ. OF A LIGHT, LOW-CALORIE BEER, OR 4 OZ. OF A DRY WHITE WINE NO MORE THAN 2-3 TIMES A WEEK.

RULE NO. 11: DON'T USE SUGAR OR SUGAR SUBSTITUTES. DO NOT USE CREAM. DO NOT USE WHOLE MILK. AVOID ICE CREAM.

RULE NO. 12: AVOID FLOUR-BASED FOOD SUCH AS MACARONI OR NOODLES.

RULE NO. 13: AVOID DELICATESSEN MEAT SUCH AS SAUSAGES, SALAMI, AND OTHER FATTY MEATS.

RULE NO. 14: AVOID RICH DRESSINGS, BUTTER, MARGARINE, OR OILS, OR ANY KIND OF SHORTENING FOR COOKING, SPREADS, OR DRESSINGS. DO NOT BINGE ON PEANUT BUTTER. LIMIT YOURSELF TO ONE SLICE OF BREAD PER DAY. ALL FISH OR FOWL MUST BE SERVED WITHOUT SKIN AND CAN EITHER BE BROILED OR BOILED. CHOOSE FRESH AND FROZEN FISH OVER SHELL FISH.

RULE NO. 15: JUICE FAST THE 1ST WORKING DAY OF EACH WEEK.

RULE NO. 16: HAVE ONE VIGOROUS WORK-OUT FOR 15-20 MINUTES DAILY.

And there you have it. When you take a good look at it, you have all of your favorite food groups to choose from on your Take·Charge·Keep·Trim Diet:

1. Fresh fruits and fruit juices.

2. Fresh raw vegetables and vegetable juices.

3. Green vegetable combinations and vegetable soups.

4. Whole grains.

5. Starchy carbohydrates.

6. Low-fat dairy products.

7. Salads and dressings.

8. Legumes as a protein option.

9. Nuts and seeds.

10. Fish, chicken, or turkey as a protein option.

A SAMPLE MENU FOR THREE DAYS

DAY 1: **BREAKFAST**
6 oz. fresh fruit juice
Fresh fruit salad
½ cup low-fat cottage cheese

LUNCH
6 oz. tomato juice
Fresh raw garden vegetable salad with many varied
    combinations
1 slice whole grain bread

DINNER
6 oz. tomato juice
Fresh raw garden salad
Baked potato without butter or salt
Chinese vegetables with tofu or chicken

DAY 2: **BREAKFAST**
6 oz. fresh fruit juice
Fresh fruit salad
7 almonds

LUNCHEON
6 oz. fresh carrot juice
Fresh raw garden vegetable salad
1 cup vegetable soup
1 slice bread

DINNER
6 oz. fresh carrot juice
Fresh raw garden vegetable salad
Steamed broccoli-zucchini combination
Corn on the cob

DAY 3: **BREAKFAST**
6 oz. fruit juice
Fresh fruit salad
½ cup low-fat cottage cheese

LUNCH
Fresh fruit juice
Fresh fruit salad
Non-fat yogurt or low-fat cottage cheese ½ cup

DINNER
6 oz. tomato juice
Fresh raw garden vegetable salad
1 cup vegetable soup
Organic bean tostado OR
4 oz. fresh fish with ½ cup brown rice

What if I don't feel quite right while I'm on the diet? What should I do?

The Del Mar Diet is carefully planned out to provide substantial food nutrients. Thousands of nutrition-conscious patients have reported success with this program. It is not uncommon to describe some symptoms of detoxification while juice fasting or cleansing. Please review the risks of the cleansing diet and how to correct them.

Once you reach your desired weight, go back to the original Del Mar rhythm diet. Stay with it for the rest of your life. Enjoy the benefits of looking great and feeling marvelous.

9: CONCLUSION

Now that you are looking trim and healthy, you are to be congratulated. Being fit to do, to get up and go, to create , to love, and to enjoy the benefits of life, indefinitely prolonged, is your reward. What you have accomplished is only the start of something wondrous. Let's face it, there are two phases to success. The first is getting there. Then, when you arrive, you realize it takes some skill to stay there.

And that's par for the course. Anything that gives you longlasting pleasure must have an enduring influence on your lifestyle. So what does it take?

I can ask you to dedicate yourself to this diet. But will you? I can direct you to pay more than lip-service to the importance of self-responsibility and daily self-nurturing. The question is, are you willing to do it?

First off, you have to take charge of your life. You must dig in, get down into the trenches, and modify your lifestyle. There is effort and dedication involved in achieving optimal health. You need will power, determination, and courage. Your strength of character, and good judgment count.

You also need the emotional stability that comes from cleansing, which is ordinarily obscured by an unwholesome body chemistry.

THE PREVENTION OF DISEASE IS SUPERIOR TO CURE.

The plain and simple truth is that the best way to prevent disease is for you to learn how to stay well. You will need a program to combat chronic fatigue, heart disease, cancer, high blood pressure, depression, degenerative illness, stress, and other nutrition-related disorders. When you create the habit of daily wellness, you are at a very positive state of mind, body, and spirit.

Remember, many so-called diets, remedies, miracle drugs, and panaceas will come and go. Not so with the Del Mar Diet. Why? Because the natural principles for sustaining optimal nourishment and the fundamental actions to prevent dis-ease will always remain the same. A consistent, fun-loving, relaxed attitude, a daily commitment to physical fitness, satisfying hard work, nutritional balance, emotionally fulfilling relationships, and the satisfaction from believing in yourself, will most certainly be the sound foundation for your well·being.

The 21 Day Del Mar Diet is your prescription to optimal nutrition. Where do you go from here? I have written THE COMPLETE 21 DAY DEL MAR DIET to serve as your ultimate wellness program. It is your step by step formula for optimal health. It will expand upon your knowledge of nutrition. It hits the basics of cleansing, detoxifying, and maintaining, your mind, spirit, emotions, and lifestyle, as well as your body. Follow it carefully and it will keep you well.

ABOUT THE AUTHOR

Dr. Meltzer is a pioneer and leading authority in the field of holistic health in California today. He was the first physician to enter the private practice of Preventative Medicine in Southern California. In addition to his thriving practice he is director of the North County Holistic Health Center in Del Mar.

Dr. Meltzer completed his conventional medical training graduating Phi Beta Kappa from the University of Pennsylvania School of Medicine. He then spent three years specializing in surgery at the University of California. His search to find solutions to our societies rapid decline in quality health led him into the field of natural healing.

Since then Dr. Meltzer has become nationally renown for his innovative natural healing techniques. It was early on in his career that Dr. Meltzer discovered that the great majority of illness, dis-ease, fatigue, depression, anxiety, indigestion, upper respiratory infections, flu, allergies, back problems, insomnia and the like could be prevented.

Teaching people how to stay well became an integral feature of his program. In his international private practice Dr. Meltzer has successfully treated more than 15,000 patients throughout the United States, Mexico, Central America and South America.

He has written the Del Mar Diet to give you the freedom of optimal health. Currently Dr. Meltzer is Professor and Dean at the Graduate School of Holistic Health and Clinical Nutrition at the University of Humanistic Studies in San Diego. There his students are earning Masters and Ph.D. degrees before joining the work force as New Age health professionals.

TAKE THE NEXT STEP

Now that you are experiencing the high of the 21 Day Del Mar Diet you will be happy to know that there is more to come.

The ultimate and most comprehensive health program has been compiled in the **Complete 21 Day Del Mar Diet.**

In this book you will get the

21 Day Del Mar *Emotional Diet:*
to acquire the habit of happiness.

The 21 Day *Mental Diet:*
to take charge of your life.

The 21 Day *Physical Diet:*
to charge up your sexual vitality.

The 21 Day *Lifestyle Diet:*
to balance your lifestyle.

The 21 Day *Spiritual Diet:*
to strengthen your spirit.

All in all you will look great and feel terrific.

Also, Dr. Meltzer offers exciting one and two day seminars, every 6 weeks on the 21 Day Del Mar Diet.

(coupon)

Send $12.95 for the Complete 21 Day Del Mar Diet (plus $1.05 for postage and handling).

Name _____

Address _____

City _____ Zip _____

Telephone: Home (_____)_____ Work (_____)_____

Send check or money order *only.* No cash please.

Mail to: **Dr. Know•How Publications**
1011 Camino del Mar, #234
Del Mar, California 92014

Allow 6-8 weeks for delivery.

☐ I am interested in attending Dr. Meltzer's workshops on the 21-Day Del Mar Diet. Please send information.

INTERESTED IN A CAREER AS CLINICAL NUTRITIONIST OR TOTAL HEALTH PRACTITIONER?

The University for Humanistic Studies
in conjunction with
The North County Holistic Health Center
Barnet G. Meltzer, M.D., Dean

Offers unique degrees:
M.A. CLINICAL NUTRITION
M.A. CLINICAL HEALTH EDUCATION
PH.D. CLINICAL HEALTH EDUCATION

FEATURING:

• The first complete graduate training in Holistic Health and Practical Nutrition in the United States;

• Distinguished faculty of Leading Holistic Health Practitioners, Professionals, Physicians, and Nutritionists from San Diego, the leading "Holistic Health Center" in the United States;

• Personalized supervision to acquire marketable skills of the expert health practitioner;

• Experiential learning to maximize the professional excellence of your services;

• Comprehensive, humanistic, innovative curriculum for maximum career opportunities;

• Specialized training to work in the "Physician of the Future" office or your own clinical setting as a health awareness specialist;

• Access to the Network of Health Professionals for job placement.

MAIL TO:
ADMISSIONS OFFICE
THE UNIVERSITY FOR HUMANISTIC STUDIES
1011 CAMINO DEL MAR, #234, DEL MAR, CA 92014 • 452-7792

I am interested in learning more about The Clinical Nutrition and Clinical Health Education Programs. I would like:

☐ An appointment to discuss programs and enrollment.

☐ A brochure and application packet describing the program. Enclosed is $1.00.

☐ A visit to class without charge or obligation.

Name _____

Phone: Home (_____)_____   Work (_____)_____

Address _____

City _____ State _____ Zip _____

Best time to be reached by phone is: _____

Comments _____
_____
_____